Ethics in Midwifery

For Mosby:

Publishing Manager: Inta Ozols
Project Development Manager: Mairi McCubbin
Project Manager: Jane Shanks
Design Direction: George Ajayi

Ethics in Midwifery

Shirley R Jones MA, RGN, RM, ADM, Cert Ed (FE), Teaching
(Midwifery), Supervisor of Midwives
Principal Lecturer/Supervisor of Midwives, School of Women's Health Studies, Faculty of
Health and Community Care, University of Central England in Birmingham, UK

Foreword by

Andrew Symon RGN RM MA(Hons) PhD
Clinical Research Fellow (Midwifery), Maternity Unit, Perth Royal Infirmary, Tayside
University Hospitals NHS Trust & The School of Nursing & Midwifery, University of
Dundee, UK

SECOND EDITION

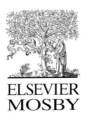

ELSEVIER
MOSBY

EDINBURGH LONDON NEW YORK OXFORD PHILADELPHIA ST LOUIS SYDNEY TORONTO 2000

MOSBY
An imprint of Elsevier Limited

First published 2000
    Reprinted 2004, 2005

ISBN 0 7234 3172 8

British Library Cataloguing in Publication Data
A catalogue record for this book is available from the British
Library

Library of Congress Cataloguing in Publication Data
A catalogue record for this book is available from the Library
of Congress

Note
Medical knowledge is constantly changing. As new
information becomes available, changes in treatment,
procedures, equipment and the use of drugs become necessary.
The author, contributor and the publishers have, as far as it is
possible, taken care to ensure that the information given in this
text is accurate and up to date. However, readers are strongly
advised to confirm that the information, especially with regard
to drug usage, complies with the latest legislation and
standards of practice.

The Publisher

ELSEVIER your source for books,
journals and multimedia
in the health sciences
www.elsevierhealth.com

Working together to grow
libraries in developing countries

www.elsevier.com | www.bookaid.org | www.sabre.org

ELSEVIER   BOOK AID   Sabre Foundation
            International

The
publisher's
policy is to use
paper manufactured
from sustainable forests

Printed in China

Contents

Foreword

In today's maternity services ethical issues are everywhere, and yet there is often a poor understanding of how practitioners deal with them. Many qualified midwives, while asserting that they are ethical in their work, might be hard pressed to define what this means in practice. An ethical approach is often assumed, as if practitioners are somehow socialised in such a way that ethical practice becomes second nature. This is a mistaken approach. It ignores the complexity of contemporary maternity care, and disregards the changing emphases between the pregnant woman and those who work within the health service. It also overlooks important developments in health care law.

In recent years there has been a drive to provide choice and promote autonomy for pregnant women. In a world with unlimited resources, such a drive would be relatively uncomplicated. In today's comparatively cash-constrained health service, restrictions are placed on the scope for achieving autonomy and exercising choice. The time available for discussions with each pregnant woman is limited. What do midwives do when faced with limited resources or conflicting choices?

This revised edition provides an accessible account of the theories used in ethical discussions, and then presents a series of case studies. These require the reader to decide how practical problems may be dealt with in an ethical manner. This combination of the theoretical and the practical will provide the reader with a sound basic understanding of ethical concepts, and an appreciation of how different people may approach a given clinical situation. While ethics is seen by some as a theoretical issue, to be debated in classrooms and conferences, the everyday import of ethical decision-making means that the theory–practice gap needs to be bridged. This book will help the reader to do this. Using role play in the classroom to enact the case studies may help students to become more aware of the different approaches that may be adopted.

Maternity care is a multi-disciplinary process. It also requires practitioners to involve the woman and her family as much as possible. Midwives are involved in clinical areas as diverse as per-conceptual counselling, antenatal screening, intrapartum care, intensive care of the neonate, and even termination of pregnancy. The exercise of maternal choice has led to requests for home births, water births, and caesarean births. Inevitably, people approach these complex areas with different views.

Something as mundane as a midwife deciding how she organises her workload may have ethical dimensions. With limited time to accomplish a series of antenatal visits, what does she do if one woman requires more of her time than she had anticipated? Is the benefit to this one woman offset by the detriment caused to the others who many receive less attention?

There is scope for conflict in many areas of midwifery. Personal opinions may make it difficult for a midwife to provide effective care. This may be most apparent in the case of termination of pregnancy. While a midwife has the option of notifying a conscientious objection to involvement in this procedure, doing so may pose practical difficulties, not least in terms of employment prospects.

The developing role of the midwife is addressed in the section 'Ethical dimensions of the midwife's role'. As part of, or in addition to, clinical duties, midwives may be involved in education, counselling, advocacy and research. The vital significance of an ethical approach to these areas is covered in this new edition. The implications for midwifery of developments in health care law are also stressed throughout the book. What, for instance, are the midwife's legal rights/legal duties in relation to third trimester terminations? How should midwives deal with the question of surrogacy? Whose interests are being followed when there is a discussion concerning the withdrawal of treatment from a severely ill baby? Just as ethical questions arise every day, so, too, are legal issues of daily importance.

All midwives, whether newly qualified or with years of practice under their belts, must keep pace with the many developments in health care. Practitioners must ensure that the requirements of professional and legal accountability are met, and must keep pace with developments in research-based clinical practice. Those new to the profession have to learn to be aware of the ethical considerations that will arise each day of their working lives. Society is changing too, and the expectations of the general public are high. All of these have an ethical dimension, and an appreciation of how to approach ethical questions becomes ever more important.

In many cases there are no simple answers, and Shirley Jones has identified areas where additional discussion may be of benefit. The combination of theory, case studies and suggestions for such further debate in this new edition will be a great help to all those involved in midwifery. I commend this book to students of midwifery, their educators, and those involved in clinical practice.

Preface

The intention in writing this book is to assist in the education of midwifery students, before and after registration, while not excluding other healthcare students. It may also be of use to others involved in the education and training of midwifery students, such as clinical midwives and lecturers. It is hoped that it will be particularly useful to those who feel threatened by the inclusion of ethics in the curriculum, if only to highlight examples and explain certain principles; however, it is not intended that this should be a definitive work.

Where to include ethics in the education programme is debatable. It could be argued that it is a basic need of the students and that, as such, it should feature as a large component at the beginning of training. It would be correct to say this of anatomy, physiology, sociology or even psychology; they are equally important for different reasons. The author considers it more worthwhile to thread ethics through the whole course, starting with the basic principles of everyday practice – such as accountability and confidentiality – working through to more sophisticated principles at appropriate stages of training. However, now that midwifery education is delivered in institutions of higher education, commonly in a modular format, this is not possible.

The book is arranged in two sections. Section 1 consists of the ethical theory, giving the background to the possible reasons for certain ethical decision-making. It then establishes the link between ethical theory and practical application and analysis, by considering the ethical dimensions of midwifery practice. Section 2 consists mainly of six case studies, in separate chapters, with relevant questions and discussion points surrounding these questions.

Each chapter has 'Further discussion' material and lists suggested reading which some readers may choose to pursue, in addition to the references. By using these case studies it is envisaged that readers will be able to apply the ethical theory from Section 1. The case studies have been ordered according to the perceived needs of students; for instance, it is assumed that the principle of confidentiality will need to be addressed before consideration of aspects of euthanasia, therefore 'Confidentiality' appears first and 'Withholding or Withdrawing Treatment' is last. Further information regarding the case studies can be found at the beginning of Section 2 and a glossary of terms used has been included to aid clarification. The characters used in the case studies and illustrative examples are not intended to depict any particular race or social class; names having been selected at random.

Readers will also find that the author has made use of some situations that are not purely midwifery, but have an obstetric bias; no apology is made for this as, in practice, these are often the areas of most concern to students and qualified midwives. This was, in fact, requested by midwives canvassed by the author at the start of the original work. There are also some situations that are non-health care but which serve to highlight or clarify the principles, without creating a confusion of issues.

The intention of this book is that it should be used according to the needs of those running the courses, or the desires of the individual who wishes to access it.

Redditch, 2000   Shirley R. Jones

Acknowledgements

I would like to thank my husband, Alan, and my mum, Dilys, for their help and support in producing the final manuscript. I also wish to thank all those people who read the first edition, thus requiring a second edition to be written.

Section 1

Ethical theories and dimensions

1

Introduction

(Note: Midwives, in this text, should be considered to be male or female; generally, feminine pronouns have been used only for ease of writing, except in Chapter 7 where the midwife is male.)

Midwifery students are embarking on an adult academic course, perhaps for the first time, and as adult learners must be responsible for their own learning. They should be self-directed, taking an active part in seeking, through their own and their peers' efforts, to broaden their knowledge; they should receive tutorial assistance that is tailored more to their individual needs. The students come to the course with a wide variety of backgrounds and experiences. In the case of post-registration students there are some similarities in professional experience, whereas pre-registration students' experiences are often very different. The differences can be used to broaden the outlook of the group as a whole and to give different perspectives on various issues, if students are given the chance to discuss freely.

When in the clinical areas, the students have to learn to identify the ethical issues, consider the possible actions that could be taken, then select the appropriate course. In the interests of safety, as these situations often need decisions to be made quickly, it would be more acceptable for the public – and less threatening for the students – to simulate situations in the classroom. This could be done by role play but it does not necessarily require practical simulation; the author's choice would be to use carefully constructed case studies. These can then be used individually or in small groups, with feedback to a larger group if appropriate, or main group discussion if numbers are not prohibitive.

If the ethics, or ethics and law, module of the reader's course is to be assessed, then written work could be practised around the cases, perhaps using the questions as a basis for formulation of an answer plan. Undertaking this activity may encourage additional reading including the consideration of newspaper articles, women's magazines and television programmes, not only 'known' texts. This may well highlight the tendency for one-sided views to be reported by the media.

It is common practice among many lecturers in midwifery, but by no means all, to start everything with a definition. The author will continue this practice by defining the title of this piece of work: *Ethics in Midwifery*. On first hearing the word 'ethics' many people believe they know what it means but would then have difficulty explaining it. Looking to a parallel profession, Gillon (1990, p. 90) explained medical ethics, briefly, as:

> ...*the critical study of moral problems arising in the context of medical practice.*

Although the power bases in medicine and midwifery are different and therefore cannot usually be substituted directly for each other, it would seem reasonable for our purposes to substitute midwifery for 'medical' in this definition. In doing this it is necessary to consider what is meant by 'moral problems'. These should be interpreted as problems involving moral values: the rights and wrongs, the 'oughts' and 'ought nots' of our practices. Perhaps a clearer explanation was given by Wilday (1989, p. 176), when she explained it as being '... the study of the underlying reasons for deciding what is best in the face of conflicting choices', there seems little need to try to improve this explanation. The best, as used here, includes both prudential and moral considerations. It may be considered prudent, for instance, to inform a woman that she may require a caesarean section for a particular complication; moral considerations, however, would suggest that she be given sufficient information, and opportunity to question, in order to give or withhold informed consent.

Anyone who is not familiar with a midwife's sphere of practice may understandably question the need for ethics at all in the educational programme. Many people think that doctors make all the decisions and so midwives would rarely face conflicting choices; however, midwifery is a parallel profession to obstetrics, and its members may be concerned with or about the dilemmas presented by conflicts in a wide range of issues:

◆ Preconception care
◆ Genetic counselling

- Genetic engineering
- Fetal medicine
- Infertility
- The reproductive revolution
- Screening for fetal abnormality
- Termination of pregnancy
- Contraception
- Care of abnormal babies
- Care of preterm babies
- Care of 'damaged' or dying babies
- Care of disabled mothers
- Care of dying mothers (including life support)
- Care of very young mothers
- Incest
- Child abuse
- Advice and care throughout pregnancy, labour and the postnatal period.

Midwives are governed by a professional body which provides information and guidelines relating to their rules and codes of practice and conduct. Doctors also have a number of codes and declarations that guide their practice, and it is always possible that conflicts will arise precisely because each profession is practising what they think their code requires of them.

REFERENCES

Gillon R 1990 Teaching medical ethics: impressions from the USA. In: Byrne P (ed) Medicine, medical ethics and the value of life. John Wiley, Chichester
Wilday R J 1989 Ethics in midwifery. Midwives' Chronicle

2

Ethical theory

IS ETHICAL REASONING PART OF EVERYDAY LIFE?

It seems obvious that ethical reasoning is an essential component of life if we choose to live in society with other individuals. The completely amoral individual is a very rare specimen; therefore the great majority of people are capable of recognising moral dilemmas and conflicts when they arise. They are recognised as a part of life, irrespective of a commitment to solving them – or success in doing so. In most situations people act intuitively if their upbringing and general socialisation have laid down good principles and values. There are situations, however, when conscious practical decisions need to be made, which are not intuitive. For example, when buying a bottle of shampoo, people would prudently select one suitable for their own or their families' hair type(s), but morally they may consider buying a brand on which animal testing has not been used. Likewise, when buying food, some may consider the use of genetic modification to be a threat to health and therefore to be avoided.

There are, of course, more serious situations, such as the teenager with a drug-addicted friend (see p. 13), the relative or neighbour who suspects someone of child abuse, or the person who drinks and drives. It could be argued that, at the time of driving while under the influence of alcohol, the driver is not completely rational (this surely is why it is inadvisable) and therefore is not actually choosing to commit this bad action. Another consideration is that if motorists have driven to wherever they are drinking without making adequate provision for the return journey, then the choice was made either when leaving home or when ordering or accepting the drinks that caused them to be over the limit.

WHAT IS ETHICS?

Ethics is the application of the processes and theories of moral philosophy to a real situation. It is concerned with the basic principles and concepts that guide human beings in thought and action, and which underlie their values. As philosophy divides into various branches, so too does ethics; it would appear to have three accepted parts:

Meta-ethics (ethics)

This is moral philosophy conducted at the most abstract level and it concerns the nature and status of moral thought and the language used: determination of what is meant by 'good', 'bad' or 'happiness', how we know that one decision is better than another, discovering reasons for moral judgements (Purtilo 1993).

Ethical/moral theory

This attempts to formulate a procedure or mechanism for solving ethical problems. Most of today's adults, as schoolchildren, learned formulae for solving mathematical problems; it could be suggested that the majority felt that they were of little use to them – purely a means of psychological torture that mathematics teachers inflicted on them! It is probable that many people have used very few of these formulae since adolescence, unless working out areas for carpets and curtains, or percentages. The reason for this, surely, is the irrelevance of some of them in the everyday lives of most people; after all, how often do *you* need to find the area of a pyramid?

Ethical problems are obviously different. They remain with us throughout life in various forms; they require decisions to be made – sometimes urgently – that will have consequences other than a tick or cross in a mathematics book. It could, therefore, be seen as essential to find a formula that can be drawn on whenever such a situation arises. The modern label for this approach is 'normative ethics'. Some contemporary philosophers, however, reject the need for formal theories which can then be applied to every situation, or a list of principles that should always be referred to. They prefer to develop the moral sensibilities of individuals so that they can discern the rights and wrongs as they arise, and within the circumstances surrounding them. This viewpoint is called 'particularism'.

Practical ethics

This deals with the specific everyday issues that occur in life generally, and also in defined areas such as medicine and business. Everyday issues cannot be divorced from the more defined issues, as people do not shed their personal moral codes (for daily living and the interaction between human beings) on entering a surgery, ward or office. This point applies to patients and staff alike; therefore, these moral codes form a core within the specifics of the defined area, in which there are issues that the average citizen would not encounter on a regular basis. Implementation of *The NHS and Community Care Act 1990*, however, created a less obvious definition between medical and business ethics in some areas. The change within the National Health Service meant that, instead of being one large multi-faceted service, it comprised a number of purchasers and providers working on behalf of the consumer (previously known as the patient or client). Business strategies were involved and therefore medical and business ethics became entangled in some areas.

The following example indicates the distinctions between the three forms of theorising outlined.

A shopkeeper discovers that a seven-year-old boy has stolen a packet of sweets; he considers this to be bad behaviour and therefore unacceptable. The shopkeeper then has to decide whether the child should be chastised with no further action, whether the child's parents should be informed for them to be aware of the misdemeanour and deal with it themselves, or whether the police should be involved as this is a juvenile crime.

◆ This is a practical situation, where the incident is happening – a decision must be made (*practical ethics*).

◆ Reference to the shopkeeper's moral principles, values or theory could determine any decision about what action to take. For example, if the shopkeeper considers that it is wrong to steal and all cases of stealing should be punished, then the matter may well be referred to the police (*ethical/moral theory*).

◆ This is the part that, rather than help the shopkeeper decide on a course of action, would consider what was meant by bad behaviour or crime (*meta-ethics*).

WHAT IS A MORAL ISSUE?

According to *The Oxford Dictionary of English*, an 'issue' is 'an important topic for discussion'. It would probably be fair to say that an issue is an important topic on which the majority of people will have an opinion. Opinions will vary – otherwise there is no real issue – and may be based on different values and beliefs; it is this variance that leads to dilemmas.

So, what is a 'moral issue'? It would appear to be an important topic relating to the rights and wrongs of everyday living; for example, the value placed on life would involve routine dealings with other people, views on abortion, euthanasia or capital punishment. It could also relate to the extraordinary events that occur, such as civil or international armed conflict.

Many problems have an obvious moral dimension and some reveal moral issues on closer inspection. However, Johnson (1990) warned of the possibility of people, once aware of medical ethics, analysing every clinical decision for moral issues; some might call this 'over-ethicising'. It was also Johnson's opinion that confusion arises between ethics and etiquette, in that social convention can be mistaken for moral principle; indeed, it has been suggested that, until fairly recently, the majority of doctors believed that medical ethics, as a subject, dealt primarily with issues of professional etiquette. Johnson gave, as an example, the practice of patients being referred to consultants only by a general practitioner (GP), failure to comply with this practice being against etiquette not ethics. In many areas this practice regarding referrals has changed in midwifery, as there are direct referral opportunities for midwives. However, there is still evidence in practice of the confusion between ethics and etiquette.

WHAT IS A MORAL DILEMMA?

Campbell (1984, p. 2) described a moral dilemma as a situation where:

> ...one is faced with two alternative choices, neither of which seems a satisfactory solution to the problem.

This is accepted by others, including Johnson (1990) and Purtilo (1993), who qualify it further by stating that the alternatives are 'apparently equal'. In a way, encountering a dilemma could be considered similar to facing crossroads, or a forked road, with inadequate directions:

> A driver has some idea of where he wants to get to; he would also like to arrive in the quickest time but with the least number of hazards on the way. In the absence of a map, written instructions or adequate signposting he has to make a decision – but will it be the right one?

Obviously, the result in this situation is not so crucial as one involving the treatment of a person, be it medical or social treatment. The example given is not a moral dilemma, it is merely a simplified indication of the basic problem. The shopkeeper in the earlier example could be seen to be in a similar situation, with three possible routes to follow.

The moral dilemmas that midwives face may not be any greater than those faced by others, just different. They are governed professionally by the United Kingdom Central Council for Nursing, Midwifery and Health Visiting (UKCC), whose *Code of Professional Conduct* (UKCC 1992) states, in the first two of 16 points:

> *As a registered nurse, midwife or health visitor, you are personally accountable for your practice and, in the exercise of your professional accountability, must:*
>
> *1 act always in such a manner as to promote and safeguard the interests and well-being of patients and clients;*
>
> *2 ensure that no action or omission on your part, or within your sphere of responsibility, is detrimental to the interests, condition or safety of patients and clients.*

Even considering situations in which one might have to take account of these two moral requirements indicates the real possibility of dilemmas emerging. An example of a moral dilemma faced by midwives could be as follows.

A primiparous woman is admitted in established labour. She has a birth plan which states that under no circumstances will she give consent to an episiotomy. This aspect is discussed with her and she maintains her stance. During the second stage of labour progress is slow but positive; however, the perineum remains thick and rigid. This is explained to the woman but she maintains her position regarding episiotomy. As time progresses the fetal heart shows signs of slight distress, to the point where most midwives would consider episiotomy to be the action of choice, but still the woman withholds consent. The midwife could either continue and hope that the fetus will survive (obviously notifying appropriate personnel) or she could perform the procedure without consent in order to protect the fetus. If she carries out the episiotomy without consent, she could face a claim of battery against her. Neither is the ideal solution. (Maternal versus fetal rights are discussed in Chapter 8.)

It is important to remember that, although everyone comes into contact with health professionals at least once in their lives, they do not all work within this sphere. It may therefore be useful to consider the moral conflicts and dilemmas that people might face outside their working lives. Imagine yourself as the central figure in the next example.

Jenny has passed her driving test and has an old car in which she and her three flatmates travel to their college. She and her friends have acquired tickets for a particular idol's concert in London. The group cannot afford the train fare but, if Jenny is prepared to drive, they can afford the petrol between them. Jenny agrees to this. On the morning of the concert, as they are preparing to leave, Jenny receives a telephone call from her mother to say that her grandmother has been taken to hospital and is seriously ill.

In Jenny's place what do you do? Do you go to the hospital and thereby break a promise and disappoint your friends who were relying on you? Or do you continue on the outing and neglect your grandmother and parents?

Another example could be what a young adolescent experiences when he becomes worried about a friend's apparent addiction to drugs.

Until he became worried, the adolescent probably felt that no dilemma existed, at least with regard to his friend. The fact that he is worried indicates that he would like to do something about it. But what? He has two basic choices, each with different consequences:

CHOICE 1
Do nothing: Consider that the friend is experimenting with aspects of life in order to enable him to make the transition into a self-determining adult. Alternatively, he may consider that it is none of his business and he has no right to interfere.

CONSEQUENCES

◆ The friend soon decides that this is not for him and gets on with his life. (If it has reached the point where our subject is concerned, then this is an unlikely outcome.)

◆ The friend becomes increasingly antisocial as a result of his addiction, possibly engaging in criminal activities to support his habit.

Or, more dramatically:

◆ The friend dies from continued drug abuse – either by developing disease(s) through his lifestyle, or by overdosing or using unclean drugs.

CHOICE 2
Tell the friend's parents so that advice can be sought in time.

CONSEQUENCES

◆ The friend is furious at the breach in friendship (i.e. privacy). He continues to use drugs but has nothing more to do with the 'sneak'. Our subject is not only without his best friend, he is no longer on hand to care for him and get help if needed.

◆ After the initial trauma of being found out by his parents, the lad is thankful that his friend sought help for him in time.

This situation highlights that neither of the choices can be considered completely satisfactory – hence the adolescent's dilemma. Basically should he do nothing and lose his friend, either to a traumatic lifestyle or even through death, or should he take action and lose his friend through betrayal of trust? Either way it would appear that he will lose out. A similar dilemma could occur where an adolescent girl suspects that her friend has an eating disorder.

Beauchamp & Childress (1994) describe two forms of moral dilemma: one form is where there seems good reason to support both performing and not performing a particular act, as in the case of the woman who refused the episiotomy; the other is where the particular action is considered by some to be right and by others to be wrong. This would include cases such as a woman, with a known abnormal fetus, making a decision regarding abortion, or the decision regarding feeding and hydration in cases of persistent vegetative state, as in the Tony Bland case (Airedale NHS Trust v Bland 1993). They also indicate that not all philosophers accept that moral dilemmas exist; these philosophers are monist, believing that all actions should be governed by one supreme duty, 'good will' for example. Immanuel Kant was one such person. He believed that all actions should be performed out of a sense of duty and right reason, never through inclination; thus intentions rather than outcomes were judged and no dilemma regarding choice existed.

WHAT IS A MORAL CONFLICT?

On first consideration, it could be assumed that conflict and dilemma are roughly the same. However, Johnson (1990) made it clear that it is actually the *conflict* between moral principles or obligations that often causes the *dilemmas*; he indicated two types of such conflict, one being the conflict within a principle, such as autonomy. Even if we accept autonomy as a moral value which should be promoted and protected, whose autonomy is most important? That of the midwife or the client? The second type is where two separate principles conflict. Here we can consider again our previous case of the labouring woman refusing an episiotomy that could protect her baby; the midwife has an obligation to value the life of the fetus but also to consider the interests and well-being of the woman.

Hopefully it is obvious that moral conflicts and dilemmas occur in everyday life, not just in specific areas such as medicine and midwifery. As stated previously, they are situations of uncertainty in which people find themselves facing choices; the more difficult it is to predict the consequences of an action, the greater the dilemma. In Jenny's situation (p. 12), perhaps compromise is possible – a visit to see her grandmother on the way to London. Compromise, however, is not always possible. How do you compromise between life or death when your choice of actions may lead to one or the other result?

HOW DO WE RESOLVE THE DILEMMAS – DO WE NEED ETHICAL THEORIES?

It was stated above that ethical theory is intended to create a mechanism with which to solve our moral problems; but is it needed? People with no background in the study of ethics also have to make their decisions. Some everyday decisions would appear to be made intuitively or practically, some with a great deal of 'heart-searching', according to personal beliefs and values. It could be suggested that very little formal, ethical theorising occurs. Generally, people would state that it is a matter of instinct, intuition or conscience and, for some, that it is dependent on circumstances. When it comes to the decision-making of a midwife about a client, or a doctor about a patient, there are legal aspects to be considered. Those people determining the legalities will no doubt consider the theoretical stances; one should therefore have a basic understanding of what these are based on.

The variety of theories that have been developed indicate the fact that philosophers cannot agree which is the most appropriate. In fact some, the subjectivists, would suggest that theories are unnecessary. They say that, as beliefs about morality cannot be true or false, there is no way of determining a correct way of living or acting; therefore no mechanism can be constructed. Norman (1988) quoted Bertrand Russell as stating that when two people disagree about values, there is no difference in objective truths, merely a difference in taste. Norman explained that Ayer & Stevenson developed Russell's view into a theory known as 'emotivism' in which feelings and attitudes play a part, as opposed to 'descriptivism' which is based on facts.

In normative ethics, generally, two major theories are considered and these will therefore be outlined. The author would then like to consider the possibility of an alternative.

ETHICAL THEORIES

UTILITARIANISM

Utilitarianism is the most prominent of the consequentialist ethical theories which has, in its purist form, a monist belief in the principle of utility. It is believed that all human beings have one thing in common: they seek pleasure and avoid pain. Individuals therefore pursue those activities that will, in the end, at least bring them pleasure and avoid those that will cause them pain. If this is true of all individuals, then a moral individual should have regard not only for their own pleasures and pains, but also for those of others. When making choices they should seek to maximise pleasure and minimise pain for all involved. Thus the general principle on which utilitarianism is based is that a moral action is that which creates the greatest happiness for the greatest number. This principle has a certain appeal at a basic level because, whatever our moral stance, most of us take some account of the probable effects of our actions on others, but a number of criticisms can be raised. However, before considering these, it is necessary to distinguish between the two forms of utilitarianism available: act-utilitarianism and rule-utilitarianism

Act-utilitarianism

This is the classic or traditional form supported and developed, for instance, by Bentham, Mill and Sidgwick in the eighteenth and nineteenth centuries. In this form of utilitarianism every single action is judged by its consequences.

The principle is simple and easy to grasp, as every action is assessed in terms of the benefit it will produce: the greater the degree of anticipated benefit, the greater the chance that the act will be right. It is a method of seeking answers to questions in an objectively calculable way, the only acceptable solutions being those that create maximum good. Efficiency is often sought by decision-makers, and act-utilitarianism can provide this too, in that conflicting interests can be compared and assessed in terms of their capacity for producing good.

Rule-utilitarianism

This modification of act-utilitarianism assesses an act according to moral rules, the right rule being that which would produce the maximum benefit. Therefore, instead of individual actions being assessed according to the principle of utility, they are assessed according to moral rules of conduct to enable them to comply with the principle of utility. This means that an act is right if it falls under the right rule; the rule is right if general observance of it would maximise utility. There is the need to determine the consequential differences in order to determine the validity of the rules, but with caution to prevent the rules from becoming too specific, and therefore ridiculous, or in fact creating a slide-back to the act itself.

Some criticisms of utilitarianism

It is necessary to consider whether the claims on behalf of utilitarianism are justified. It is considered to be simple and calculable in terms of utility, forward looking to the *possible* benefits and *probable* costs. However, the apparent simplicity of assessing everything in terms of benefit disappears when benefit itself is examined closely. How do you measure utility, or usefulness? It is possible that everyone would have a concept of these words, but would they have the same concepts and the same priorities? When considering the benefit principle, it is difficult to assess whether this is achieved by creating a lot of benefit for a few people, or a little for a greater number of people.

It is also preferable to know whose utility should be considered. People would presumably start with themselves, but then would also need to consider their families, as individuals can have a major effect on each other's lives. People also affect, or are affected by, those they work with, those they live near, and the nation of which they are a part; if benefit is to be maximised, very soon people could justify personal responsibility for the world. How should the benefit of different people(s) be compared?

As Glover (1988, p. 63) rightly said: 'The problems are obvious'. Total happiness could mean increasing the levels of pleasure of existing people, or it could be increasing numbers of happy people. If increasing numbers means increasing the size of the nation (population), this could cause a decrease in the level of individual happiness, by overcrowding, inadequate food, poor health, and therefore increased mortality and morbidity rates. Some, including Bentham, say that animals should be included, but even if considerations are restricted to human beings, which generations matter? When contemplating the happiness of future generations, it is not certain what life will be like for them and, therefore, it is not possible to anticipate their pleasure accurately.

Utilitarianism can place unreasonable demands on individuals, considering everyone as equal when clearly they are often unequal, particularly with regard to responsibility. A woman with children would be considered to have different responsibilities to a woman with no dependants, whereas someone whose job includes policy-making has responsibility for the greatest good for an even greater number of people. Also, while considering communitarian outcomes, the individual may be required to sacrifice personal happiness in favour of the majority.

There are moral objections to consequentialism, in that the *means* may include acts of dishonesty or injustice. For non-utilitarians such acts would be against their codes of conduct, as this could mean that 'local' misery is created in order to achieve 'global' benefit. This can create conflicts with individual integrity and has little regard for the protection of individuals. Take, for example, the following situation from Smart & Williams (1988, pp. 98–99); it is not a midwifery situation, but one that highlights the difference between the utilitarian and the deontologist.

Jim is a botanist on expedition in South America. He finds himself in a small town where 20 Indians are tied up ready for execution, following acts of protest against the government. The captain, Pedro, having explained the situation, offers Jim a guest's privilege of killing one of the Indians himself. If he accepts, as a special mark of the occasion, the other Indians will be freed. If he refuses, then there is no special occasion and Pedro will have them all killed as previously planned.

If Jim is a utilitarian he will have no qualms about carrying out the execution; after all, to lose one life in order to save 19 produces a better consequence than losing all 20 lives. If he is a non-consequentialist then the possibility of committing murder, regardless of the consequences, would be against his moral integrity. If Jim killed the one, he would be responsible for that one death. What would his responsibility be, however, if Pedro carried out the 20 executions? Would he be responsible for the deaths of the other 19? This would be negative responsibility, which a utilitarian may well consider appropriate in this case. A non-utilitarian, however, would not accept this, believing only that Jim is responsible for his own actions.

There can be definite practical problems with utilitarianism: the difficulty of predicting all the possible consequences of an action, and difficulty in accurate prediction of those considered. How, in fact, are the consequences planned for? What time span is considered? How broad is the thinking and how many alternatives are to be considered? If we are seeking to arrive at a decision then there is often no time for protracted pondering.

DEONTOLOGY

Deon is the Greek word for duty, and, as the term suggests, deontological theory considers duty to be the central issue, as opposed to teleological considerations of deontology, which consider that everything has been created by God to serve humankind. Deontologists believe that what is good in the world stems from people doing their duty. They consider duty first, regardless of the consequences, with the notion of happiness fitting in where, and if, it can. Perhaps this can be illustrated by considering the men who, despite personal risk to themselves and the knowledge that they may never return to their families, enlisted with the armed forces in the two World Wars. Whether we approve of armed conflict or not, we must assume that, at least some of those who did not wait to be conscripted, did so from a sense of duty. This duty was essentially to 'King and Country' and in the defence of their own families.

As with utilitarianism, there is more than one theoretical version in deontology; in fact there are three. These theories not only compete with utilitarianism, but also with one another.

Rational monism

This moral theory was constructed by Immanuel Kant, who claimed not to be creating a radically new moral theory, rather he thought he was formalising how people already thought. In his view the only moral actions are those performed through a sense of duty. One's duty is to do what is rational and moral, all actions proceeding from a 'good will' will be moral in this sense. To help identify which actions are or, more properly, which actions *are not* moral, he offered his theory of the 'categorical imperative'. The categorical imperative is about 'oughts' and 'ought nots', and is very definite and decisive: duty for duty's sake controlled by one's conscience (Warnock 1998).

The hypothetical imperative, on the other hand, is less definite, using terms such as 'if ... then' and 'in order to ...', 'If you want to do or achieve *X*, then do *Y*' or 'in order to achieve *X*, do *Y*'. For Kant this was not definite enough. His first moral test of an action was by universalisability, that is consideration of an action in terms of the effect if everyone acted in the same way, in the same circumstances (Warnock 1998). These two examples may help to see this law more practically:

I keep my promises. If everybody did, would it be right?

Clearly, in this case, it would (depending on the promises), but:

I do not agree with paying National Insurance payments, therefore I shall refuse to pay them. If everyone refused to pay, would it be right?

In this case, regardless of personal views about this charge, it would not be right as there would be no money for the provision of services.

Kant's second test involved the consideration of the autonomy of people:

'Act in such a way that you always treat humanity, whether in your own person or in the person of any other, never simply as a means, but always at the same time as an end' (Kant, in Palmer 1999, p. 113)

Doctors are expected to be deontological, in that that they are expected to abide by the Laws of Humanity as formulated by the

Declaration of Geneva. Similar expectations of nurses, midwives and health visitors are held, as determined by the UKCC in the codes of professional conduct and practice and the midwives' rules and code of practice (UKCC 1998). These are not scientific laws, nor are they positive laws of which a legal system is comprised, rather they are natural or moral laws.

'Traditional' deontology

This has a strong religious basis, with a belief in God and the sanctity of life. Moral duties are taken from the Ten Commandments and it would seem logical to assume that devout Christians, and those with other beliefs where the Commandments in general and the sanctity of life in particular are featured, would consider this theory to be the basis of their moral decision-making. As can be seen, the Ten Commandments form a good basic model of 'dos and don'ts' and do not create moral conflicts. The avoidance of conflict occurs because each addresses a different prohibition or obligation; therefore, it is possible to abide by them all simultaneously.

> *Thou shalt have none other Gods before me.*
> *Thou shalt not make thee any graven image…*
> *Thou shalt not take the name of the Lord thy God in vain…*
> *Keep the sabbath day to sanctify it…*
> *Honour thy father and thy mother…*
> *Thou shalt not kill.*
> *Neither shalt thou commit adultery.*
> *Neither shalt thou steal.*
> *Neither shalt thou bear false witness…*
> *Neither shalt thou desire thy neighbour's wife…*
> *(The Holy Bible, Genesis 5)*

Intuitionistic pluralism

Unlike rational monism, this version of deontology advocates no supreme principle, rather it suggests that there are several moral rules or obligations to be followed which are of equal importance. There is always the possibility of rule conflict though, so how is this resolved? Ross considered seven prima-facie duties which he believed reflective people would accept (Gillon 1986), and these were to be carried out unless specific situations proved prohibitive:

1. *Duty of fidelity* This involves keeping promises, being loyal and not deceiving. Is this what we expect of our Government as well as individuals?
2. *Duty of beneficence* The obligation to help others.
3. *Duty of non-maleficence* Not harming others, which is more stringent than any other duty.
4. *Duty of justice* To ensure fair play.
5. *Duty of reparation* An obligation to make amends.
6. *Duty of gratitude* To repay in some way those who have helped us (owed to special people such as parents); this also includes loyalty.
7. *Duty of self-improvement*

The problems arise when these duties also conflict. For instance, in order to keep a promise or be loyal to a friend, you have to be disloyal to or offend a parent; here there is conflict between the duties of fidelity and gratitude. As no one duty has an automatic lead, there is no hierarchy, so how do people decide how and when to override one duty by another? In the Jewish and Roman Catholic religions, in Kant's view and to some extent in the British legal system, there is a system whereby such conflicts are resolved; it is called 'casuistry'. This system of case-based reasoning had fallen into disrepute for many years but has been revived over recent times (Beauchamp & Childless 1994, pp. 92–93). The system allows for disentanglement of the conflicting rules and reordering them in accordance with the situation. Despite the pitfalls created by conflict of duties, it is interesting to note that medical ethics has found this pluralistic model attractive; for midwives it is apparent in the UKCC *Code of Professional Conduct* (UKCC 1992). Arguably the most common problem arising for midwives, from the 16 '*duties*' laid down in the Code, is the conflict of autonomy:

[...]

   1 act always in such a manner as to promote and safeguard the interests and well-being of patients and clients; [...]

   6 work in a collaborative and co-operative manner with health care professionals and others involved in providing care, and recognise and respect their particular contributions within the care team.

The problem that arises usually involves conflict between the autonomy of the woman and that of the midwife, but also between the midwife and other healthcare professionals (see Ch. 7 on Autonomy and consent).

ANOTHER ALTERNATIVE?

It was stated above (p. 8) that some philosophers – particularists – reject the need for formal theories which can then be applied to every situation. They prefer to develop the moral sensibilities of individuals, enabling them to discern the rights and wrongs as they arise and to act with the flexibility required of the specific situation. The principle of truth-telling may again be a good example here. If, according to deontological belief, we have a duty to tell the truth at all times, what happens on the occasions when telling the truth will cause offence? If to tell a lie would create no harm, but would prevent causing offence, that could be a better course of action – without having mentally to conduct an act-utilitarian experiment to see which course produced the greatest amount of good.

Particularism gives this flexibility (McNaughton 1988). It does not say that we can ignore morality, rather that we educate children, through all the avenues of socialisation, to recognise the right action to take in the situation in which they find themselves. This education would undoubtedly change its style and content according to the age and development of the child. Some moral guidance would be offered in the form of commands to a young child, as a means of protection, until the child is mature enough to be discerning.

From the midwifery point of view, an avenue of socialisation could be the inclusion of moral rights and principles in the educational programme, which should then be applied in practice, while ignoring the traditional duty-based and consequentialist theories. Another possibility would be to develop an eclectic theory, as has been achieved with models of care, taking the best aspects of a number of theories. Elements of Kantian ethics and pluralism appear to fit with a client-centred approach to caring and the duty of care. However, aspects of utilitarianism are worthy of consideration, especially within the National Health Service, where the greatest benefit must be achieved for the greatest number of people, but not at any cost – the ends do not always justify the means.

Seedhouse (1998) writes about act-deontology and rule-deontology, either of which could be seen to be eclectic developments. However, for those who are just beginning to grasp an understanding of ethical theory, it is probably wiser to learn about and evaluate the traditional, more straightforward, theories first, before delving into the newer approaches.

REFERENCES

Airedale NHS Trust v Bland 1993 1 All E R 821
Beauchamp T L, Childress J F 1994 Principles of biomedical ethics, 4th edn. Oxford University Press, Oxford
Campbell A V 1984 Moral dilemmas in medicine, 3rd edn. Churchill Livingstone, London
Gillon R 1986 Philosophical medical ethics. John Wiley, Chichester
Glover J 1988 Causing death and saving lives. John Wiley, Chichester
Johnson A G 1990 Pathways in medical ethics. Edward Arnold, London
McNaughton D 1988 Moral vision. Blackwell, Oxford
Norman R 1988 The moral philosophers. Clarendon Press, Oxford
Palmer M 1999 Moral problems in medicine. Lutterworth Press, Cambridge
Purtilo R 1993 Ethical dimensions in the health professions, 2nd edn. W B Saunders, Philadelphia, Pennsylvania
Seedhouse D 1998 Ethics. The heart of health care, 2nd edn. John Wiley, Chichester
Smart J J C, Williams B 1988 Utilitarianism for and against, Cambridge University Press, Cambridge
UKCC 1992 Code of professional conduct for the nurse, midwife and health visitor. UKCC, London
UKCC 1998 Midwives rules and conduct of practice. UKCC, London
Warnock M 1998 An intelligent person's guide to ethics. Gerald Duckworth, London

SUGGESTED ADDITIONAL READING

Bowden P 1997 Caring, gender-sensitive ethics. Routledge, London
Garrett T M, Baillie H W, Garrett R M 1993 Health care ethics: principles and problems. Prentice-Hall, London
Mason J K, McCall Smith R A 1994 Law and medical ethics, 4th edn. Butterworths, London

3

Ethical dimensions of the midwife's role

In recent years attempts have been made to reclaim our overall midwifery role, having gradually lost it during the period of medicalisation. Midwives and women's groups have blamed the doctors of the time who persuaded politicians and local providers of the need for 100% hospital provision for childbirth. The doctors concerned were generally obstetricians, whose teachings were heard from the mouths of the newly qualified doctors who maintained the philosophy within the hospitals and spread the teachings through the community as they passed into general practice. General practitioners who had supported women and midwives in their continuance of home birth (within certain criteria) found themselves marginalised by their new partners who were reported to say such things as 'If you want childbirth at home then you will have to cover the on-calls 24 hours per day, 7 days per week', and so on (personal experience). According to Chamberlain et al (1997), however, it was women who led the movement into hospital, through fashion and the availability of analgesia, and the professionals followed on. Regardless of who was responsible for past changes, in reclaiming their position in the childbearing arena midwives realise that this does not mean regression. Rather it is a matter of reclaiming what was good and, with reference to evidence and research, moulding it to meet the needs of women and midwives in the twenty-first century.

The overall midwife's role can be subdivided into separate aspects: practitioner, adviser, counsellor, advocate, friend, educator and, more recently, researcher. Within these roles lie responsibilities that are outlined in the various documents produced by the United Kingdom Central Council for Nursing, Midwifery and Health Visiting (UKCC). In general terms, these responsibilities include:

◆ Maintaining and improving the safety of mother and baby
◆ Providing quality care and unbiased information and advice which are research/evidence-based
◆ Educating and training students to be able to join the profession and provide the service with the same level of responsibility as their more experienced colleagues, that is being 'fit for practice' and 'fit for purpose' (UKCC 1999, p. 34).

This does not mean that students should be able to practise, from the outset, as if they have five years of experience. Although experienced midwives may acquire extra responsibilities related to grading and management posts, the basic responsibilities do not alter with experience. A major responsibility, upon which most of the others depend, is that of professional updating, thus continuing to be 'fit for practice' and 'fit for purpose' (UKCC 1999). In order that midwives can give up-to-date information and provide care that is research/evidence-based, it is essential that they read current professional literature. Midwives today are very fortunate as there is a variety of midwifery literature on the market; they do not have to rely on the *Midwives Chronicle* alone. There is also a wealth of material available in journals which relates to the health service more generally, or allied professions, where articles pertinent to midwives as health carers are published. It could be advantageous for midwives and doctors in relevant specialties to read one another's journals. This could lead to a broadening of views and some healthy debates over various interpretations of the content. Accepting someone else's interpretation about research findings, without reading the report and formulating a personal opinion, could lead to a 'Chinese whispers' misinterpretation.

Midwives in current practice have always had a responsibility to update or 'refresh' themselves, unlike their nursing and health-visiting colleagues for whom this became a reality only in 1995, with the start of the Post-Registration Education and Practice (PREP) initiative. This change, which is being phased in for midwives, is very flexible. It allows the practitioner to make use of a wide variety of updating methods, not just attendance at a residential refresher course, or attendance at any available study days with National Board approval, as some midwives realise that five years is almost up and they do not have seven certificates to present to their Supervisors! Now reading the literature counts. A midwife can spend a morning in a university library reading a variety of journal articles, followed by an afternoon writing an account of what has been learned from the reading. The hours spent on the whole exercise will count towards five days or 35 hours of PREP (UKCC 1997), if the evidence is in their professional profile.

Occasionally concern is expressed within the profession that some midwives may not undertake their updating through the new system. However, although it is the responsibility of each midwife to fulfil the UKCC requirements, managers will be aware of some of the updating undertaken, unless it is all taking place in the midwife's own time. As managers are responsible for providing a high-quality, contract-specific service within set resources (Williams & Hunt 1996), they should be aware of how their workforce is developing. The additional safeguard within midwifery is the statutory supervision of midwives. Through this system, the Supervisors of Midwives should be assisting midwives to assess their own needs, and they should be assessing that the needs are being met. If there is no proof of updating, the midwife is in breach of the above-mentioned codes and rules by which she is governed.

Having responsibilities is similar to having moral duties within deontological theory, and we can be called to account for our short-comings, within the profession, our employment and in civil law. The term commonly used for moral responsibilities and actions in professional settings is ethics; the ethical dimensions of the midwife's role will be considered under the headings of the subdivisions mentioned earlier.

PRACTITIONER

Midwives have become increasingly aware of the term 'duty of care'. Many are encouraged to learn about such aspects of common law as they undertake educational courses. They also read the excellent journal articles by authors such as Bridget Dimond and Andrew Symon. Sadly, some midwives appear to be interested because they have a fear of what they consider to be increasing litigation. There seems little evidence of consideration of the underlying ethics on which common law is based. Codes of practice and conduct indicate the ethical framework within the practitioner's field. Upholding these ethical codes results in us practising within our professional rules and, therefore, within the law. Failure to uphold the codes may result in a charge of misconduct, that is, failing to conduct oneself in a professional and, therefore, ethical way. The professional rules and codes within which UK midwives practise do not state explicitly that we have a 'duty of care' (see Ch. 6 on Accountability). However, in the *Guidelines for Professional Practice* (UKCC 1996) under the heading 'Duty of care', it is stated that we have a 'duty to care'. This explicit ethical statement is based on the implicit statements throughout the rules and codes documents (UKCC 1992, 1998), which indicate the manner in which this duty should be carried out.

As practitioners, how do midwives carry out this duty? It could be said that it is a matter of conscience for the individual midwife and, to a point, this seems reasonable. However, there are times when one person's conscience will allow them to act differently to others. This could result in midwives exhibiting a poor general attitude to clients or relatives. It could also result in occasions when verbal or physical abuse is used (Jones 1996), or other generally unacceptable practices are evident, such as telling lies, stealing from clients or divulging personal information about clients. As an individual's conscience is developed through various aspects of upbringing, socialisation and experience, there is no set standard by which its application can be judged. Therefore, although reliance on conscience might be sufficient in most cases, particularly in urgent situations, it is flawed and does not always help in times of dilemma.

To assist with decision-making in difficult situations, individuals could resort to the ethical theories, such as deontology and utilitarianism (see Ch. 2). Although these theories are ancient in their origins, they have been adapted over time and their tenets still have relevance today, with standards by which our actions could be judged. It could be argued that upholding a pluralist's belief in the duties of beneficence, non-maleficence, fidelity, justice, reparation, gratitude and self-improvement is a laudable manner in which to live one's life or conduct one's midwifery practice. It could be argued, also, that elements of Immanuel Kant's theory are laudable: that we should not use anyone as a means to someone else's ends, therefore upholding the principle of autonomy as being essential. This view is being more openly expressed in midwifery. These comments suggest that midwives are innately deontological in some way. This may be the case at an individual's 'bedside' or on occasions where a midwife has a small number of clients for whom to care. However, it becomes more difficult where greater numbers of clients are involved. A community midwife with 12 postnatal visits and an antenatal clinic has a resource problem: lack of time. The midwife in charge of a ward of 25 antenatal and postnatal women, plus the babies, also has a resource problem: all resources, including staff and time, have to be divided between the number for whom she has a duty to care. She may be able to follow deontological duties and principles with regard to the clients to whom she has allocated herself, but she cannot do this for all of them. Here she is more likely to be utilitarian in her approach, trying to achieve the best that she can for everyone. The utilitarian belief that the end justifies the means is also observed, although not consciously, in that staff may not take their breaks in order to get the work done. When staffing levels are low, there is an increase in the utilitarian approach, with aspects of care such as support for breastfeeders receiving less attention for the few, in order to carry out more of the less time-consuming activities for the many.

The *Code of Professional Conduct* (UKCC 1992) appears to be eclectic: it has elements of various theories embedded in it, and so has taken away the theorising for the midwife. However, midwives should analyse the sections to ensure that they are observing them adequately and can be secure under scrutiny, should they be called to account for their actions or omissions.

Midwifery is moving slowly towards supporting autonomy in its clients. The publication of the report *Changing Childbirth* (Department of Health 1993), which sought to increase the choice, continuity and control for childbearing women, had an ethical basis, particularly involving the principles of autonomy and justice. Many midwives saw this document as the key to a future in which midwifery was regained for women and midwives; where autonomy and choice were the rule rather than the exception. However, despite the development of a variety of good pilot schemes, financial constraints have prevented many of them from continuing or expanding. Many midwives are sad at the loss of this golden opportunity, although not all midwives were completely in favour of the recommendations of this report. Some considered that the required changes would affect their personal lives, while others did not want to foster autonomy in the clientele. This view was not necessarily related to wanting to retain power and control, but to genuine paternalism: these midwives fervently believed (and presumably still do) that they and their professional colleagues had greater knowledge and therefore knew what was best for those in their care (see Ch. 7 on Autonomy and Consent). While on an academic level we might strongly support autonomy and discourage paternalism, there are times when paternalism is required, such as when a woman is out of control. It might be needed only fleetingly, but it can be useful and, in cases such as this, is used to enable the woman to regain control. It is probable that all midwives could be accused of using a 'soft' paternalism on occasions, as we have all used powers of persuasion to achieve our aims.

Midwives have a legal and ethical duty to provide quality care and to ensure and maintain safety. Difficulties arise, however, when there are staff shortages. Midwives are forced to move from a more deontological stance of upholding various duties and principles for each individual, to a more utilitarian approach to all within broader principles. It could be argued that NHS Trusts are unethical in their demands of midwives during such shortages. Not only do the midwives feel under undue pressure to achieve the impossible in the given time, but they are also aware that, under scrutiny, they could be accused of failing in their duty of care. Although, in a civil suit of negligence, it is the Trust that would be vicariously liable, it is still the midwife who is left feeling morally bruised at providing substandard care.

Midwives, like other healthcare workers, may face personal dilemmas when compliance with the woman's choice would lead to self-compromise for the midwife. This could be a situation where a woman who is labouring at home is using illegal substances to assist with pain relief. Alternatively, it could be when a client has decided to undergo termination of her pregnancy on the grounds of fetal abnormality. In the first example there is nothing that the midwife can do, other than maintain safety in areas over which she has control. There is no issue of public safety to warrant a breach in confidentiality by notifying the police. The second example, however, may be different, depending on any previous notification of a conscientious objection to involvement in termination of pregnancy (see Ch. 8). In neither of these cases is the midwife entitled to exhibit a judgemental attitude (UKCC 1992, 1996).

EDUCATOR

Midwives in most areas have a two-pronged role in education, in that they are responsible for educating parents and various students. Mothers, their partners and sometimes other family members, usually require assistance to develop skills and acquire knowledge in the areas of baby care and health promotion. As knowledge gives power, education is also about empowerment (Collington 1998). The degree of help depends on the experience of the family in question.

Today's midwife will usually aim to work with the mother to determine and fulfil her individual needs, thereby acknowledging client autonomy. It would be unusual to experience the paternalism of earlier years, which insisted that all women, whatever their background or experience, were required to undergo the same educational pattern of demonstration, then practice under supervision (for every practical skill), before being allowed to care for their babies. This aspect of the role requires continued updating by the midwife, as wrong or inadequate information could lead to a charge of negligence.

An area of heated debate within the profession centres on educating women with regard to making up formula feeds and sterilising equipment. One side of the argument is that more emphasis on breastfeeding and less on bottle-feeding would be best practice; therefore, educating breastfeeding mothers in practices related to bottle-feeding is thought to be counter-productive (Jamieson 1997), as is the practice of having prepared feeds on view in postnatal areas. It is thought by protagonists on this side of the argument that, should the mother wish to give a bottle at any time, or when she needs to know how to sterilise equipment, she can read the information for herself on the relevant packaging.

Those on the other side of the argument, who might still be avidly in favour of breastfeeding, feel that there is an element of coercion rather than free choice. They believe that some women who have chosen to bottle-feed, or even those with human immunodeficiency virus (HIV) or taking potentially harmful medication, where they have been advised not to breastfeed, may be made to feel bad mothers. This is achieved as they have to slink into a designated room or, worse still, find an already harassed member of staff to fetch a bottle. Another area for concern on this side of the debate is that, should a breastfeeding mother resort to bottle-feeding for any reason and her baby becomes ill, through feeds made up wrongly or equipment improperly sterilised, the midwives could be seen to be at fault. Part of their duty of care is to foresee some of the problems that a new mother may encounter, and teach and advise appropriately. Some women cannot read well enough to interpret instructions on boxes. Others who can read well may make errors when trying to make-up a feed for a very distressed baby. These errors could happen even where the education has taken place, although this is less likely and the midwives would not be at fault.

The other prong of education relates to students and inexperienced staff, who are many and varied. There are those undertaking work experience in their school education programme, various nursing students, healthcare assistants, medical students, obstetric and paediatric house officers and, more specifically, student midwives. This section will concentrate on student midwives.

Midwives are the gate-keepers of their own profession; they are ethically and legally responsible for maintaining, wherever possible, the safety of mothers and babies. They are almost completely responsible for teaching skills, and they share the responsibility with academic colleagues for the teaching of knowledge and attitudes to students. They have the power to prevent the qualification of inappropriate students – where repeated clinical assessment shows them to be unsafe or exhibiting unacceptable attitudes. This could be seen as a negative responsibility, one that, fortunately, does not need to be exercised very often. A positive ethical responsibility requires that midwives ensure that their students practise up-to-date skills and apply current theory to practice.

Failure to teach and assess students adequately creates new generations of inadequate midwives, such as a generation of midwives who are totally dependent on electronic fetal monitoring, or who are unable to define fetal position on vaginal examination during labour, or who are ineffective decision-makers. Midwives must take care not to pass on inadequacies, biases, quirks of practice and weaknesses, yet they should also avoid the tendency to produce professional clones. Many midwives will remember being trained to stand on the woman's right-hand side for every procedure, even though she might be hard of hearing on that side, or the student might have been left-handed – hardly the safest practice when considered fully. Such training also discouraged autonomous practice and assertiveness; often the latter came only with long-awaited seniority.

Occasionally students fail to achieve their theoretical or clinical learning outcomes and, although this is very difficult for them as individuals, it supports the rigour of the course which, in itself, is designed to produce safe, effective midwives who are acceptable to women and their families. On even rarer occasions, fortunately, such students become qualified practitioners, and clinicians question the educational institution as to why it passed someone who is unsafe or unfit to practice. Clinicians have the responsibility to be honest in their assessment of students and, where they feel such errors have occurred, they should look to their own accountability and that of their colleagues.

COUNSELLOR

This aspect of the role includes the provision of information and explanation, as well as listening and assisting women and their families to explore areas of interest or concern. Midwives are responsible, within their duty of care, for ensuring that the information is up to date and that they understand it themselves, in order to give explanations or answer questions. It is thought that the information should also be unbiased but, as Chamberlain et al (1997) state: 'This utopian ideal of an unbiased profession is hard to find ...', which is not surprising as the very fact of having the knowledge is almost bound to influence the informer's approach. Apart from the fact that midwives should be seen as knowledgeable practitioners, this also serves to reduce the number of professionals that women need to see. This non-therapeutic form of counselling is utilised when women are making choices between options related to care, or when being approached for their consent or refusal to screening or invasive procedures, for themselves or their neonates.

Although, in the UK, there is no absolute legal principle of informed consent (Kennedy & Grubb 1997), common sense suggests that no true decision can be made, to give or withhold consent, based on no information. Practitioners are, therefore, expected to give 'reasonable' information – that which most similar practitioners would deem suitable for decision-making. However, if a woman requests full information, the practitioner is responsible for giving as much accurate information as is possible, or finding someone who can. This is part of the duty of care and failure to fulfil this duty – at whichever level is required – could lead to a charge of negligence if harm has occurred as a result. It is, therefore, essential that midwives keep abreast of the rapid scientific and technological changes taking place.

One area of almost continual change is that of screening. No sooner have midwives learned the relevant information regarding a particular test or procedure than another appears in the frame. It is important that the midwife knows about the disease or condition being screened for, the method of screening, the time-scales involved, the format and meaning of the results, and the options open to the woman with adverse results. As the screening menu increases, so must the midwives' knowledge. From April 2000, screening for hepatitis B virus must be offered to all pregnant women in England and Wales (NHS Executive 1998), and HIV screening by the end of the year. Keeping abreast of such developments is very time consuming, but necessary.

Regardless of the legal position relating to informed consent, midwives have an ethical duty to provide sufficient information, in order to acknowledge and support the woman's autonomy. If the woman is a self-determining, rational person, then she is deemed autonomous and able to make choices; failure to enable her to do so deprives her of a moral right. Midwives often complain that their performance with regard to counselling is inadequate because of time constraints. This suggests that, unless staffing levels are adjusted in line with midwives' current and expected duties, women's rights will continue to be eroded.

Within the counselling situation, women may disclose personal and sometimes disturbing information about themselves or their families. It could be argued that the more successful the midwife is in building a good rapport, the more likely the woman is to disclose to her. She must be aware of the woman's right to confidentiality, ensuring that, unless in exceptional circumstances, as laid down by the UKCC (1996), this right must be upheld (see Ch. 5).

ADVISER

This role should be limited if practice upholds client autonomy. Clients will require information, as previously stated, in order to make their own decisions and maintain personal control. It is very tempting to offer unsolicited advice, based on our experiences and comments from other clients or colleagues. This is paternalistic and prevents, or at least delays, the development of self-determination in our clients. Those who advise and instruct, for the purpose of gaining or maintaining power, are not paternalistic, rather they are dictatorial.

There are times when clients ask: 'What would you do?'. Midwives should be careful to consider (if they choose to respond to this question) whether their answers are reflective of their personal or professional views. For instance, having given the required information, a midwife may be asked which method of anaesthesia she would choose for an elective caesarean section. The midwife, as a professional, may have a view that is contrary to that which she would choose for abdominal surgery on herself. Screening for fetal abnormality is another area where personal and professional opinions may differ. It could be argued that personal opinions should not be voiced in a professional relationship. On the other hand, midwives should not be expected to behave as professional robots. Perhaps the important point is that the midwife should make clear the stance she is taking.

Stating an opinion is not the same as offering advice, although clients could assume that it is. Therefore, midwives need to contemplate this carefully, rather than making unconsidered, 'off the cuff' comments. They are accountable for the advice they give because, although it is not intended to be directive, women may feel obliged to follow it, or they may want to please the midwife.

FRIEND

Many midwives will remember the days when they were taught *not to get involved* with their patients. The resultant aloofness was considered to be the professional approach, enabling patients and their families to feel that we were capable, trustworthy and in control. Also, there was probably an element of consideration for self-protection in this attitude. Unfortunately, the air of detachment sometimes gave the impression of being uncaring, unapproachable and 'in charge'. The notion of being a professional friend is appealing to those who support the principle of client self-control (i.e. autonomy) and is more achievable where continuity of carer is the norm. It could be argued that this level of attachment can create dilemmas regarding counselling, advising and giving bad news. However, the opposite may well be true: that a professional friendship enables both the midwife and the client to face difficult situations. It is important to be aware of the potential of a professional friendship to create a dependence, thus replacing the old controlling paternalism with a modern protective paternalism; however, used appropriately, it enables the midwife to provide advocacy and support.

There is also the potential for development of professional friendships with student midwives, particularly during long placements. Although this is generally seen as a positive move from the attitude experienced by many midwives, there is a possible disadvantage within this change. It is possible that a less detached relationship could compromise judgement with regard to objective assessment, causing greater difficulty in referring students when learning outcomes have not been achieved. Many lecturers have heard the sad lament of a midwife, similar to: 'I hate to fail her, she is such a nice girl'. Despite the terminology used, this could refer to a student of any age and is never intended to be patronising (the situation could be similar, with appropriate wording, for male students). The key to this situation is honesty. Honesty in contemplation of the safety of women and their babies and in consideration of the student's development. Acknowledgement of an aspect of the student's practice that is in need of development means that there is the potential for achievement. Failure to acknowledge the flaw in development means that there is the potential that the student will never have the opportunity to address the issue successfully. If the assessment in question is the final one, then failure to acknowledge the flaw results in a midwife being unfit to practice at the point of registration. The midwife, the clients and the service are then potentially at risk for the future.

ADVOCATE

Professional codes require that we put clients before colleagues or the professions (UKCC 1996). In academic settings where simulation exercises are used or scenario analysis takes place, there is rarely a problem with midwives exhibiting good skills related to advocacy. In similar situations in practice, however, these skills do not appear to be as polished. Something seems to happen in between the classroom discussion and the similar occurrence in clinical practice. It is possible that the tension of the real situation dulls the cues, thus preventing the midwife or student from recognising the similarity. Also, fear of repercussions – from overbearing midwives as well as doctors – appears to encourage passivity instead of assertiveness on a client's behalf. Advocacy is linked to being a professional friend and upholding the principle of autonomy. Midwives who do not rise to the challenge of being advocates for their clients, are essentially in breach of their *Code of Professional Conduct,* clauses 1 and 5 (UKCC 1992). This aspect of the midwife's role can be particularly challenging when the client refuses, or withdraws, consent for treatment which the professionals consider to be advisable or even essential to prevent morbidity or mortality. At one time, Jehovah's Witnesses and the use of blood products would be the first example to spring to mind. In recent years, however, this may have been replaced by a client's refusal of caesarean section. The midwife's role here should be one of advocate, not oppressor, despite her (understandable) personal feelings of desperation.

RESEARCHER

Most aspects of the role require the midwife to update; therefore, reading about and practising up-to-date evidence-based methods of care are essential. Also, midwives are increasingly undertaking or becoming involved in various research activities and should be familiar with the principles and aspects of moral philosophy (ethics) that should underpin a study. While it is interesting to examine the ethical underpinning of pieces of published research, it is obviously too late to be of benefit to the participants already used in those studies. However, adequate knowledge and analysis of probable and possible concerns, at the proposal stage of new research, will be of definite benefit to the participants and of academic benefit to the researchers.

Research has blossomed within the field of midwifery, as it has in all branches of nursing. In part, this was based on the need to prove the professional and academic status of our profession to medical colleagues – to be seen as having opinions of worth rather than subjective intuition. There was also a positive aspect to this growth: the desire by an initial minority of midwives effectively to challenge outdated practices. As the profession became linked to higher education, through the validation of education and training courses, initially at diploma level, it has been expected that all students would have education in types and processes of research.

Midwives who are undertaking clinical research activity have a responsibility to ensure that ethico-legal consideration is given to the proposal. Such considerations have been included in the conduct of human research since the development of the Nuremberg Code in 1947, as a response to the scientific atrocities carried out in Nazi concentration camps during the Second World War (Fabick 1995). Personal accounts of the atrocities experienced or observed by the prisoners themselves, expressed through various forms of communication during the ensuing years, suggest that consent was not sought from the subjects in these experiments. It is unlikely that those responsible for the experimentation would even have considered consent, particularly as their subjects were deemed to be non-persons. The Nuremberg Code, therefore, acknowledges the rights of people to determine what happens to them in the name of research; informed consent is considered to be absolute and, therefore, inviolable.

In 1964 the World Medical Association took forward the issue of respect for persons and observance of human rights, which includes the protection of the rights of research subjects; it produced the Declaration of Helsinki which was updated last in South Africa in 1996 (Munzorová 1998). The ethical guidelines inherent in this document favour the well-being of the individual participant taking precedence over the interests of science, researchers and society as a whole. This is in keeping with the deontological end of the theoretical spectrum, as the utilitarian perspective, based on cost – benefit analysis, is that the good for society, not the individual, should be the guiding principle.

Consent is often viewed as an ethico-legal issue, as ethical principles appear to underpin much of civil law, particularly the torts (claims of civil wrongs). Where research is concerned, however, it would be useful to consider ethics and law separately. In English law there is no requirement for fully informed consent; all that is required is a general explanation of the course of action that is intended (Montgomery 1997), with the general purpose of justifying the care or treatment proposed and of gaining the patient's trust and cooperation (Donaldson 1992). Consent, either expressed or implied, is required only for invasive procedures, where medication is given, or for procedures that require touching of the person; carrying out the treatment, having failed to obtain consent, leaves the practitioner open to a charge of battery (Montgomery 1997). It would seem sensible on the part of a researcher, therefore, to give a broad account of what the research entails and to obtain consent from the client for any invasive research being undertaken. However, not all research is physically invasive. This would suggest that, legally, consent is not required for any research involving qualitative methods.

The ethical view of consent is linked with the principle of autonomy: if the person is deemed autonomous, consent is essential in order to preserve that autonomy. For the person to be autonomous and, therefore, in control of her life, she cannot make decisions based on broad and woolly information. She needs to know what the research is about: what it is for, why it is necessary, what her actual involvement will be and for how long, who will be conducting the part of the research related to her, any known benefits or risks, and what will happen to the results? Ethically it would be expected that practitioners would obtain informed consent, but not only for physically invasive procedures.

To be satisfied that consent is informed, it is important to use clearly worded, detailed literature to reinforce explanations given (Corbett et al 1996). After sufficient time has been given for the individual to reflect on the verbal and written information, opportunity should be given for her to ask questions of those who are in a position to answer. It is inappropriate for someone with little knowledge of the study to be in a position to receive the consent; this would increase the possibility of wrong, or at least inadequate, answers being given to the client's questions. In an ideal situation the informative part of the process would be completed well in advance of the subject being included in the study, with consent being sought at the time of entry to ensure validity as far as is possible. This is a particular area of concern with regard to childbearing women and their babies (BPA/RCOG 1991, AIMS/NCT/MA 1997).

Clients are observed on a routine basis by their carers; they are observed for signs of pain and illness, or lack of the same, and for their manner of interaction with others, such as the interaction between mothers and their babies. Consent is not requested for this observation; it is part of the package of care and the findings are used to determine the care for the specific individuals. Observation techniques used in ethnographic research yield much information about those being observed, yet the purpose is to use that information initially for the researcher's benefit, not the benefit of those being observed. Although the intention and outcome might be that future clients would benefit from the research, information relating to the subjects is being recorded and used, probably with no benefit to them (i.e. non-therapeutic research). It would seem reasonable to request consent for the observation and subsequent use of the information. This, however, could create a problem with the validity of the results. The presence of an observer will make some difference in any case, but the subjects might behave very differently if they knew they were the focus of the observation (Hilton 1987), thus creating a false picture for the observer.

As the results may be affected in this way, it could be argued that they should not be used in determining any change in practice or care, which suggests that the research was a waste of resources in the first place. This creates a dilemma: on the one hand the research could be undertaken without the subjects' full knowledge, which could be seen to be deception, akin to stealing information, and could also be considered an invasion of privacy (Haddad 1996). On the other hand, the researcher could be honest and face the possibility of invalid results. There is a third possibility, if the observation is of two people together (e.g. a mother and a midwife): the observer could tell the subject that it is the other person who is being observed. Ethically, this cannot be condoned as, again, it is deception and, even if the researcher's conscience would permit this behaviour, codes of professional practice would not uphold it.

Quantitative research also creates problems related to consent, particularly with randomised controlled trials (RCTs) and, while midwives may not lead many such projects, they are often involved in projects undertaken by doctors and should be aware of the ethical aspects involved. The very nature of RCTs means that the participants do not know to which of the *treatments* they have been allocated, as such knowledge would invalidate the research (Garrett et al 1993). This essentially means that they receive information regarding the general nature of the study, but do not know what they are to receive until they have received it and the study is complete (Clark & Hunt 1994). The willing participants consent to non-specific treatments, in that they are consenting to any of the possible 'treatments', for example: the new and the old, the new and a placebo, or all three – although it could be considered unacceptable to use a placebo when an effective alternative exists (Veatch 1989, Josefson 1997). It is possible that participants are consenting based on very little explicit information about what is being used. Treatments already in use will have known side-effects; these can be outlined to the participants, but there will be limited information regarding the new treatment which, if it is a drug, may not be fully licensed (Hewlett 1996). Placebos can create problems in themselves, depending on what is used; even vitamin C can have unpleasant effects on some people, but it is uncertain how explicit researchers are regarding the use of placebos. Where double-blind trials are used, potential participants should be told that, as the researchers do not know who is in which arm of the study, they may not be able to respond quickly to changes in the person's condition (Garrett et al 1993).

Clients may feel coerced into agreeing to participate in a study. This may be related to the manner of the person attempting to recruit participants, or it may be something quite different. The recruiter may have a manner that intimidates the client, whereby she feels unable to say 'no'; linked to this may be the fear that, whatever has been said, she will not be treated justly if she refuses. It is also possible that the recruiter is very pleasant, perhaps very persuasive, and the client feels that she really wants to help her, rather than giving any consideration to herself. Something similar can occur when face-to-face interviews are used to collect data; the participants may be afraid to say what they really want to say, or they may try to please the interviewer (Rees 1995). Researchers need to be aware of their personality type and ensure that they do not use it in a coercive manner, thus taking advantage of people in their care. Williams (1995) also highlights the problem encountered in action research of whether the participant is consenting to the recruiter as a known carer or as a researcher. It is important that the researcher explains his or her role in the study, to prevent unintended deception.

Recruiting pregnant women into research studies can be fraught with difficulties with regard to consent. In each case the woman has to think of the effect on her fetus(es), not herself alone. This may create recruitment difficulties, as most women will be concerned to protect their unborn babies and will avoid involvement in any action that could put them at risk. If these women are led to believe that their unborn babies may benefit from participation in the study, they are more likely to consent to it. These women, therefore, are particularly vulnerable. Robinson (1988) stated that some of the problems in obtaining consent to research in obstetrics relates to the attitudes of some researchers towards women, where reassurance is given instead of information. Although this statement was made some years ago, verbal accounts from women suggest that, in some cases, the position is unchanged. It is widely recognised that childbearing women should be in control with regard to their care, which includes any research study in which they are asked to participate; they cannot maintain control without adequate information.

Other pressures relate to timing of the recruitment. There can be problems in the more acute setting of the labour ward, where difficulties may arise through lack of time to consider the information given, or even lack of concentration due to pain. In these cases the situation is complicated by the client's immediate need to trust in the expertise and judgement of the professionals (Tobias 1997), which is unlikely to be enhanced by the uncertainties inherent in a research study.

Some research projects require the use of information recorded in midwifery records or delivery registers; but to whom does recorded information belong? The documents obviously belong to the provider: the researcher or, in the case of medical records, to the general practitioner or hospital; however, it is the information recorded on the documents that is in question. It could be argued that personal observation and interpretation belong to the person who wrote it, whereas factual information belongs to the person to whom it relates, hence the production of laws and codes of conduct relating to confidentiality and privacy. In the case of medical records, it is usually assumed that implied consent by clients exists with regard to access by staff on a 'need to know' basis. That is, only those who are involved with caring for or treating the person need to have access to the records. This creates a dilemma where retrospective studies are undertaken. On the one hand, failure to obtain the person's permission to view and use their information could be considered an infringement of privacy; on the other hand, it could be considered impractical to attempt to contact hundreds or thousands of clients. It is probable that many of those undertaking such studies do not face the dilemma, as they do not give thought to ownership of information and consent to access to it. If they do consider it at all, they may decide that what the client does not know about will not harm her. This attitude is ethically unacceptable as it may lead to tortious practices, such as the practice of medical students undertaking vaginal examinations under anaesthesia without the consent of the women concerned (Wright 1995).

There would appear to be a gender bias in some researchers where female subjects are concerned (Robinson 1988); for this reason, many women have welcomed the development of *feminist research*. The principles involved in this type of research are commendable, including that it should be: woman-centred, woman-focussed and woman-valuing, reflexive, egalitarian and empowering; active not passive, acknowledging the expertise of women; and with women, not on women (Dobraszcyc 1995, AIMS/NCT/MA 1997).

It could be argued that those best placed to undertake qualitative research on women are women themselves, as they may be better able to understand their subjects. A similar argument could be made by the male half of society, or by different minority ethnic groups. The position becomes more difficult when gender and ethnicity come together: if research is to be undertaken on African Caribbean women and there are no African Caribbean women suitable or willing to undertake the study, would it be better to have a Caucasian woman or an African Caribbean man? Which is most important, the gender or ethnicity? Ethically, considering aspects of justice, there could be as many problems with researchers of the same gender or ethnicity, as with those where they differ. In all cases researchers may hold their own biases and stereotypes, and these can influence the interpretation of their findings. If the main aim of feminist research is to highlight women's experiences (Draper 1997), then it should be carried out justly, regardless of the gender of the researcher.

In view of the issues raised in this section, it is important that midwives play their part in ensuring that true ethical consideration is given before research is undertaken by them. They should question any research project in which they are required to assist and they should be critical in their reading of research reports before attempting to utilise it. They cannot absolve themselves from accountability to their clients by considering that ethical implications are someone else's concern; just because approval has been given by an ethics committee, does not make it watertight. Is there a formula that they can apply quickly to a study in which they are asked to participate, in order to satisfy themselves of an ethical underpinning to the study? The answer is 'yes': a midwife should consider, as a matter of conscience, whether she would be content to change places with the subject, or whether she would wish to recruit members of her family or circle of friends. If she hesitates in this exercise, then she is smart; if she is dubious, then she has more questions to ask before participating.

As has been demonstrated, there are a number of aspects to the overall role of the midwife, each bearing responsibilities. The midwife is legally and ethically accountable for fulfilling those responsibilities within the essence of the rules that govern her and the codes that guide her. It is not easy to fulfil the overall role well, particularly as each situation is different. The midwife's role is filled with challenges, and most midwives meet most of those challenges, most of the time. Midwives are remembered fondly, indefinitely, by the women for whom they have cared, despite the traumatic outcomes that some women experience. The twenty-first century will undoubtedly set new challenges for midwives and the women for whom they care; let us hope that we, and those who follow after us, can rise to meet those challenges.

REFERENCES

Association for Improvements in the Maternity Services, National Childbirth Trust, Maternity Alliance 1997 A charter for ethical research in maternity care. (draft)

British Paediatric Association, Royal College of Obstetricians and Gynaecologists (Standard Joint Committee) 1991 A checklist of questions to ask when evaluating proposed research during pregnancy and following childbirth. Bulletin of Medical Ethics October (72):5–8

Chamberlain G, Wraight A, Crowley P 1997 Home births. Parthenon, Carnforth, UK

Clark E, Hunt G 1994 Ethics in nursing and midwifery research. Distance Learning Centre, South Bank University, London

Collington V 1998 Midwives as educators: perceptions of a changing role. British Journal of Midwifery 6(8):487–496

Corbett F, Oldham J, Lilford R 1996 Offering patients entry in clinical trials: preliminary study of the views of prospective participants. Journal of Medical Ethics 22:227–231

Department of Health 1993 'Changing childbirth' report. HMSO, London

Dobraszczyc U 1995 From notes of presentation at a conference – 'Never mind the quantity – check the quality', North Staffordshire College of Nursing and Midwifery, 13 May 1995

Donaldson, Lord 1992 Re W [1992] 4 All ER 627

Draper J 1997 Potential and problems: the value of feminist approaches to research. British Journal of Midwifery 5(10):579–600

Fabick M 1995 Ethical considerations for research on human subjects. Plastic Surgical Nursing 15 (4):225–231

Garrett T M, Baillie H W, Garrett R M 1993 Health care ethics: principles and problems, 2nd edn. Prentice-Hall, New York

Haddad A 1996 Acute care decisions: ethics in action. Registered Nurse March:17–19

Hewlett S 1996 Consent to clinical research – adequately voluntary or substantially influenced? Journal of Medical Ethics 22:232–237

Hilton A 1987 The ethnographic perspective. Distance Learning Centre, South Bank University, London

Jamieson L 1997 Knowledge and skills involved in infant feeding. In: Henderson C, Jones K (eds) Essential midwifery. Mosby, London, ch 13, p 265

Jones S R 1996 Client abuse and the personal cost of accountability. British Journal of Midwifery 4(6):295–297

Josefson D 1997 US Journal attacks unethical HIV trials. British Medical Journal 315:765

Kennedy I, Grubb A 1997 Medical law, 2nd edn. Butterworths, London

Montgomery J 1997 Health care law. OUP, Oxford

Munzorová M 1998 Declaration of Helsink – really amended? Bulletin of Medical Ethics 134:2

NHS Executive 1998 Screening of pregnant women for hepatitis B and immunisation of babies at risk. HSC1998/127. NHSE, London

Rees C 1995 Survey methods in midwifery. British Medical Journal 3(12):652

Robinson J 1988 Pregnant guinea pigs; the consumer perspective. In: Bromham D R, Dalton M E, Jackson J C (eds) 1988 Philosophical ethics in reproductive medicine. Manchester University Press, Manchester

Tobias J S 1997 BMJ's present policy (sometimes approving research in which patients have not given fully informed consent) is wholly correct. British Medical Journal 314:1107–1114

UKCC 1992 Code of professional conduct for the nurse, midwife and health visitor. UKCC, London

UKCC 1996 Guidelines for professional practice, UKCC, London

UKCC 1997 PREP and you. UKCC, London

UKCC 1998 Midwives rules and code of practice. UKCC, London

UKCC 1999 Fitness for practice. UKCC, London

Veatch R M 1989 Medical ethics. Jones & Bartlett, Boston

Williams A 1995 Ethics and action research. Nurse Researcher 2(3):49–59

Williams E, Hunt S C 1996 Supervision in midwifery practice: the debate and some evidence. Offprint in: English National Board 1997 Open Learning Pack: Preparation of supervisors of midwives, module 1, offprint 3, p 42

Wright J 1995 Respecting rights. Nursing Standard 9(34):43

Section 2

Case Studies

2

Introduction to the case studies

Some pre-registration midwifery students will be embarking on an adult education course, perhaps for the first time, and as adult learners must be responsible for their own learning. Post-registration students may also be undertaking education of a more adult nature than they experienced in their initial nursing and midwifery training. They should all be self-directed, taking an active part in seeking – through their own and peers' efforts – to broaden their knowledge; they should receive tutorial assistance that is tailored more to their individual needs. Students come to their courses with a wide variety of backgrounds and experiences. In the case of post-registration students there will be some similarities in professional experience, but they bring a richness of examples to discuss. The pre-registration students will possibly be very different. These differences can be utilised to broaden the outlook of the group as a whole and to give different perspectives on various issues, if they are given the chance to discuss freely.

When in clinical areas all the students will need to learn to identify the ethical issues, consider the possible actions that could be taken, then select the appropriate course of action. In the interest of safety, as these situations often need decisions to be made quickly, it would be more acceptable for the public, and less threatening for the students, to simulate situations in the classroom. This could be done by role-play, but it does not necessarily require practical simulation; the author's choice would be to use carefully constructed scenarios as well as real case studies. These can then be used individually, in small groups with feedback to a larger group if appropriate, or main group discussion if numbers are not prohibitive. It is important to consider and avoid, with all the cases and questions, the possible temptation to say: 'It depends' or 'It's up to her/him or them' (Downie

& Calman 1987). This may occur particularly when people feel threatened and do not want to face or expose their feelings on certain subjects, especially if it is a topic that they have never openly discussed before.

It is also important, whilst acknowledging the earlier warning against over-ethicising, to avoid a tendency to fall back on clinical as opposed to ethical distinctions. This situation can be seen in midwifery practice with regard to rupturing of fetal membranes in labour. Midwives can often be heard to extol the virtues of leaving them intact; their reasoning, however, is usually clinically based rather than on the grounds of the woman's autonomy.

If the reader wishes to use these case studies with her peers, she must remember the need for a safe environment when people are expected to expose their views; she may wish to involve a tutor to facilitate the group in setting up this activity safely. It needs to be stated at the outset that everyone is entitled to their own opinions and that there may be considerable differences within the group, but also that it would be expected that there should be an honest conflict of views. Obviously sensitivity is required as some participants may well have experienced some of the situations under discussion; it is also necessary to prevent the formation of 'encounter' groups. Facilitation may also be required to tease out areas that have been overlooked or avoided; someone may be required to play 'devil's advocate' in order to achieve this.

Where to include ethics and law in the education programme is debatable. It could be argued that it is a basic need of the students and that, as such, it should feature as a large component at the beginning of training. It would be correct to say this of anatomy and physiology, or psychology also; they are equally important for different reasons. However, the author would consider it more worthwhile to thread ethics and law through the whole course, starting with basic principles of everyday practice, such as accountability and confidentiality, and working through to more sophisticated principles at appropriate stages of training. Some aspects could be studied as individual topics which would then be applied to relevant situations. This is just one view, however, and very difficult to follow in a modular system. The intention of this book is that it should be used according to the desires of the individual who wishes to use it.

The following chapters include six case studies, dealing with topics about which midwives have expressed concern (to the author): confidentiality and privacy, accountability, autonomy and consent, conscientious objection to participation in abortion, assisted conception, and withholding and withdrawing treatment of a neonate. The case studies have been constructed, based on actual incidents, to be of particular interest to midwives of all levels. For those with a deeper understanding of medical ethics, seemingly unrelated cases create fewer problems. These students are better equipped to apply the principles to various situations and can utilise nursing or medical ethics texts throughout their midwifery education. There may be many, however, who enter midwifery without such depth of understanding. For these students, personal experience has shown that it is preferable to apply the principles within the sphere of midwifery practice first, before developing the ability of application in and from other fields.

Some of the case studies that follow consider the midwife, and in one case a student midwife, and her actions, whereas others involve her with other health professionals, particularly doctors. Some cases do not focus on dilemmas specific to a midwife, but are situations in which midwives have a responsibility and should know something of the ethico-legal issues that are involved. Each case study is accompanied by the theory relating to the major issues expected to be raised. However, during consideration of the questions, particularly during any group discussion, it is quite possible that other moral issues and philosophical principles may arise; this has been anticipated to a certain extent by bringing some of the other points into 'Further discussion', and where applicable indication is given as to which other chapter may be useful.

As previously stated, the characters in the case studies and other examples used are not intended to depict any particular race or social class; names were selected at random. To consider different races, religions or social classes could possibly add a new dimension to the cases; this activity could be carried through by interested readers if they wished to consider what difference, if any, would be made.

If the ethics module of the reader's course is to be assessed, then written work could be practised around the cases, perhaps using the questions as a basis for formulating an answer plan. This may encourage additional reading including the consideration of newspaper articles, women's magazines and television programmes, not only 'known' texts. Consideration of such material may well indicate the tendency, in some cases, for one-sided views to be reported by the media.

REFERENCES

Downie R S, Calman K C 1987 Healthy respect – ethics in health care. Faber & Faber, London

5

Confidentiality and privacy of client information

Helen, a primigravida, was 27 weeks pregnant and had been admitted to hospital with possible preterm labour. Following investigation by speculum examination of the cervix, cardiotocographic monitoring, and laboratory examination of a high vaginal swab (HVS) and a mid-stream specimen of urine, the diagnosis of a urinary tract infection was made. Treatment was prescribed and Helen was advised to remain in hospital for another day while treatment started to take effect and her pain eased. The midwife and junior student midwife (Carmel), who had been allocated to care for Helen, explained the test results and suggested treatment, with which Helen was satisfied. They also took the opportunity to undertake various aspects of health promotion and parent education. At the end of her shift the midwife wished Helen well, explaining that she would be attending a study event the next day and therefore would not see her again. She and Carmel had recorded their health promotion and parent education activities in Helen's case notes.

The next morning Carmel was allocated to the same clients, along with Anna, the midwife with whom she would work for the next two shifts. At 08.45 hours Mr Fisch, a consultant obstetrician, arrived on the ward. He wanted to see his two preterm labour clients before starting his antenatal clinic. He named the women, collected the case notes himself and was directed to a four-bedded bay where he was introduced to Helen, by her full name. While Mr Fisch looked at the case notes, Carmel drew the bedside curtains, in order to create an illusion of privacy, as there were two other clients in the bay at that time. By the time the task was completed, Mr Fisch had started speaking to Helen, so Carmel remained still, virtually behind the others involved. Mr Fisch was talking to Helen about the fact that her apparent preterm labour had been stimulated by her urinary tract and vaginal infections. Carmel was puzzled as she had seen the laboratory reports the previous day and the HVS report stated 'normal flora only', which the midwife had explained to her meant no infection was detected. Yet the consultant was now talking about *chlamydia* and *gonorrhoea*, and the possible problems that could ensue, such as preterm labour, in the case of *chlamydia* (Lyndsay 1997), and in both cases serious neonatal conjunctivitis (Simpson 1997). Carmel felt that there must be some mistake, that Mr Fisch must have confused the two clients, although she had no knowledge of the other case concerned. She wanted to alert Anna but was not in a position to get eye contact with her.

Carmel became aware that Mr Fisch had finished speaking and was turning in order to leave the bedside. Helen did not speak but looked stunned and this was noticed by Anna because she asked if Helen was alright. She got no response so she said that she would be back when Mr Fisch had seen his other client. They all moved from the bedside and Mr Fisch was waiting to be directed to the other client. Carmel took the opportunity to guide Anna swiftly out of the bay, into the ward corridor, where she explained her concern. Mr Fisch had caught up with them by the time Carmel had finished and Anna conveyed the concern to him. They checked the names on the two sets of case notes and this proved that Carmel was correct. The consultant swore quietly, hesitated, then said that he would send his registrar to explain as he needed to get to his clinic now. He did not speak to his other client at all.

Anna and Carmel went back to Helen. She was very distressed about three things: what would happen to her baby, how she could have caught these diseases, and why Carmel and the other midwife had lied to her about the results of the tests.

QUESTIONS FOR CONSIDERATION BY THE READER

1. Why are confidentiality and privacy important principles?
2. Could Carmel have prevented the situation from happening?
3. Was Anna, as the qualified midwife, in a position to explain the consultant's mistake to Helen?

4. Whoever explained to Helen, would they be at risk of breaching the confidentiality of the other client involved?
5. Is there ever a time when it is acceptable to breach confidentiality?

QUESTION 1: WHY ARE CONFIDENTIALITY AND PRIVACY IMPORTANT PRINCIPLES?

To determine the importance of maintaining confidentiality and privacy, it is necessary to consider what it means. Many definitions of confidentiality are very wordy but they almost all contain the word 'trust'. Relationships in midwifery, as in all areas of health care, are centred on trust. A woman entrusts a midwife with a great deal of personal and generally private information. When she does this she has the right to expect that this information will remain confidential and private, being passed on only with her consent, in order to maintain human dignity (Purtilo 1993). Her right in this case is a moral one as there is no statutory right to confidentiality (Darley et al 1994, Mason & McCall Smith 1994). The privilege of confidentiality belongs to the client/patient and not to the healthcare professionals, as such a breach of confidentiality or privacy can lead to legal action in the civil courts (Darley et al 1994). It can also lead to criminal action, but this is not for the breach itself, rather it is for the use to which the information is put and the harm that ensues, such as blackmail letters to well known women regarding their recent abortions, following theft of a general practitioner's computer (Anderson 1996).

In the case of midwifery/medical records, however, it is not considered reasonable to seek specific consent for the passage of information between professionals caring for each woman/patient. This is covered by 'implied consent' (see Ch. 7 on Autonomy and Consent) where, in giving information that is to be recorded in the woman's/patient's file, the person is implying consent for other healthcare professionals who will have contact with her/him, to have access to this information. This, however, is considered to be on a 'need to know' basis in that only those professionals who need to know the information, in order to care for the individual concerned, will be given access to it.

Consider the ward reporting system in your unit at the shift handover: Who is present? What information is passed on? Do all those people need to know all that information? It could be suggested that this is one area where midwives fall down on the observance of the 'need to know' principle and, therefore, on the observance of the principles of confidentiality and privacy (Robinson 1996)

QUESTION 2: COULD CARMEL HAVE PREVENTED THE SITUATION FROM HAPPENING?

Mr Fisch knew who his clients were; he was introduced to Helen by name and he had both sets of case notes to check before embarking on his encounter with her. Carmel was either aware of the need to protect a woman's privacy at such times, or was at least aware of the common practice of closing curtains to give the illusion of privacy. This practice, while proper, cannot be considered anything but illusory. Conducting doctors' rounds in two-, four- or six-bedded bays, as is common in many modern hospital layouts, is only a number-reduction of the problems of such rounds carried out in the older dormitory-style Nightingale wards. In such circumstances it was common for all patients to be in their beds, curtains were drawn while each patient was seen in turn, and the conversations were heard by all except the most hard of hearing. After the visiting group had left the main ward, doors were closed but curtains were all neatly pulled back, and patients could be heard to 'play the game' by asking those on either side or opposite what everyone already knew but pretended not to: 'What did he say to you then?'

Having undertaken her task with the curtains, Carmel was polite in not trying to improve her physical position in the group, which could have created an untimely distraction. Had she been less polite, she might have been in a position to catch the eye of Anna, to signal that something was wrong. If Anna had picked up the signal, she might have tried to look at the notes to see whether she could determine the reason for Carmel's disquiet. She might have remembered the names and diagnoses or conditions of the clients as told to her at the shift handover, thus realising the confusion. However, it is more likely that she would have registered the signal and decided to speak to Carmel once away from the bed.

Another course of action open to Carmel was to interrupt the consultant and say that she thought there might be some mistake. Many qualified midwives might find this difficult, unless they were absolutely certain of an error; it is therefore likely that a junior student would find it impossible. In Carmel's case, what made it more difficult was the fact that she knew nothing of the other case; she was not in a position to know that there was an error, only to suspect it strongly, and the doctor was the person with the evidence in his hands.

Even if she had found the courage to speak up, she could not know that Mr Fisch had made a mistake until he had already given out wrong information. So, although she could possibly have stopped the proceedings and allowed the error to be acknowledged and corrected, she could not have prevented the whole problem. While it could be said that Carmel should have spoken sooner, it could be argued that, under the circumstances, as a junior student, she acted very politely and responsibly, creating awareness of the problem as quickly as could reasonably be expected of her.

QUESTION 3: WAS ANNA, AS THE QUALIFIED MIDWIFE, IN A POSITION TO EXPLAIN THE CONSULTANT'S MISTAKE TO HELEN?

It is probable that most people would consider that Mr Fisch should have returned to Helen immediately, to correct his mistake and apologise for it. He is accountable for his actions, both the initial error and the way in which he chose to deal with it. However, although he is the accountable person, he has created difficulties for his registrar, who now has to try to correct an error in which (s)he played no part. The registrar will undoubtedly apologise to Helen on Mr Fisch's behalf, but a proxy apology means very little to most people, added to which there will be a time lapse during which Helen is worried and upset unnecessarily.

Anna has a dilemma: if she follows Mr Fisch's decision and waits for the registrar, then Helen continues to suffer unnecessarily. Alternatively, if she explains to Helen, she could be seen to have acted against the decision of the consultant who, at least for this episode within Helen's pregnancy, is the lead professional. The situation should be analysed and considered in terms of possible consequences in order to determine the best course of action. In practice, of course, Anna will have to do this very quickly. Mr Fisch did not give permission for Anna to deal with the problem: he nominated someone else. It could be argued that he did not say that she could not deal with it; he may not even have considered that possibility in the heat of the moment. However, as he made a positive decision to send the registrar, that is the course of action which should, theoretically, be followed.

Practically, however, this leaves an untenable situation. Helen is very upset about three points in particular. First, she has unnecessary worries about the condition of her fetus, which she already thinks of as a baby, as do most women in pregnancy. There is probably no worse problem for most pregnant women than concern about fetal well-being. Second, she is concerned about how she has contracted these sexually transmitted diseases. She knows her own sexual history and there could be aspects of this that cause her to feel responsible and therefore guilty for the situation she now faces. She could be worried about telling her partner: if she tells him, this could be the end of their relationship; if she does not, he could already be or become infected. Probably there is nothing for her to feel guilty about, so her thoughts turn to her partner: he must have been unfaithful to her! This thought could lead to further anxiety. Third, she thinks that Carmel and the midwife caring for her the previous day have lied to her. They did not just conceal the results until the consultant came, they actually told her that the HVS was clear.

Despite Mr Fisch's decision, the registrar would not be able to attend quickly enough to prevent increasing emotional harm to Helen. Anna cannot allow the situation to continue; she has a duty of care to Helen which is stronger than her duty to protect a professional colleague with regard to his carelessness or to follow his expressed decision (see Ch. 6 on Accountability) (UKCC 1992). This is, after all, an ethical matter, not one where the clinical judgement of an obstetrician is essential. If Anna decides that she has to deal with the matter immediately, then she faces her next dilemma: exactly what it is that she is going to explain.

QUESTION 4: WHOEVER EXPLAINED TO HELEN, WOULD THEY BE AT RISK OF BREACHING THE CONFIDENTIALITY OF THE OTHER CLIENT INVOLVED?

The results that Mr Fisch gave to Helen were from someone else's case notes. This means that very sensitive information about one person, who will be called Susan, has been given to another. Worse still, the person who received the information was another client, not even someone involved in caring for Susan. When the consultant gave the information, he did not know that he was passing on someone else's information; the breach, therefore, was not intentional but an accident. Nevertheless, it has occurred through carelessness which, from Helen's point of view, might be considered negligence.

At the point when the consultant left the ward, Helen did not know that she had been given Susan's information, nor did Susan know that her information had been given to Helen. Once Helen is told what has happened, apart from her possible claim regarding negligence, she will become aware that someone else has got the diseases that she was told about. She will not be told the name of the other woman, but she will probably guess that the information relates to the other woman whom the consultant was going to see when leaving her. It is possible that Susan is one of the other clients in Helen's bay. While the healthcare professionals cannot be held responsible for Helen determining who this other woman is, it could be argued that she would not have been able to do this without the initial error.

It is possible that some readers may think that, once Helen's mind has been put at rest, there is no further concern. They may regard her knowledge of the sensitive information as no worse than in the normal ward-round setting, as described above, where clients hear what is said to those around them. This may be so but, ethically, it would be more correct to say that the ward-round practice regularly infringes clients' privacy and should be changed, rather than accepting the infringements as routine and unavoidable.

Once they have dealt with the error from Helen's point of view, consideration needs to be given with regard to Susan. Someone will have to tell her the results and implications of her tests. Will they also tell her that her results, albeit anonymous, were given to someone else? In practice this is unlikely to happen, partly to prevent more upset than is necessary, but mainly in the hope of avoiding litigation. In theory, it could be argued that a wrong has been committed and should be put right at whatever cost; therefore, Susan should be told what has happened.

QUESTION 5: IS THERE EVER A TIME WHEN IT IS ACCEPTABLE TO BREACH CONFIDENTIALITY?

Midwives, as with nurses and health visitors, are guided by the *Code of Professional Conduct* (UKCC 1992), clause 10 of which states:

> *'Protect all confidential information concerning patients and clients obtained in the course of professional practice and make disclosures only with consent, where required by the order of a court or where you can justify disclosure in the wider public interest.'*

This is further explained in *Guidelines for Professional Practice* (UKCC 1996, p. 27), where 'public interest' is interpreted as:

> *'...the interests of an individual, of groups of individuals or society as a whole, and would cover matters such as serious crime, child abuse and drug trafficking or other activities which place others at serious risk.'*

However, the Code also states that the practitioner must be able to 'justify disclosure'. In the situation under discussion, Anna would be justified in explaining the situation to Helen, particularly as she would not directly be identifying Susan. Mr Fisch, although not governed by this particular code of conduct, would be governed by the General Medical Council's document *Professional Conduct and Discipline: Fitness to Practice* (GMC 1993), which states:

> *'Doctors therefore have a duty not to disclose to any third party information about an individual that they have learned in their professional capacity, directly from a patient or indirectly.'*

It has previously been stated that healthcare clients have the civil right to expect that the principles of confidentiality and privacy should be upheld. There are times, however, when there are competing rights, or when the rights of one individual conflict with the rights of another. In this case there was no initial conflict of rights which justified Mr Fisch divulging the sensitive information to Susan. His unjustified action could therefore be considered a violation (Beauchamp & Childress 1994). At the point where Anna was faced with Helen in a distressed state, there were conflicting rights: Helen's right to a proper explanation of the cause of her distress and Susan's right to protection of her information. Anna could be seen to be justified in indicating that the results related to another client, even though Helen might be able to determine her identity; this would therefore be considered an infringement (Beauchamp & Childress 1994).

Purtilo (1993) lists the legal exceptions to standard practice with regard to maintaining confidences:

◆ in emergencies
◆ where patients/clients are incompetent or incapacitated
◆ when protecting third parties
◆ when required by law
◆ when hospitalising psychiatrically ill patients.

FURTHER DISCUSSION

There are two terms that cover similar areas but which are considered by some to be separate – confidentiality and privacy – both of which can be infringed or violated.

Infringement or violation of confidentiality

An infringement of X's confidentiality occurs only if the person to whom X disclosed the information in confidence, fails to protect that information or deliberately discloses it to someone without X's consent. (Beauchamp & Childress 1994, p. 418)

To put this into context:

Shirley (the course tutor) tells Lorna (a colleague) that she is pregnant but that she does not want to tell anyone else yet. If Lorna tells another colleague then this is deliberate disclosure, a violation of confidentiality. Also, Shirley's group of students could discuss with Lorna the fact that they are worried about Shirley, as she looks pale, tired or ill. If Lorna did not want the students to be concerned unnecessarily, and therefore explained the reason for her colleague's appearance of ill-health, she is still guilty of the infringement of confidentiality.

Infringement or violation of privacy

...only a person or institution to whom a patient grants information in a confidential relationship can be charged with violating confidentiality. (Beauchamp & Childress 1994, p. 41)

For example, if a person gains unauthorised access to a hospital records department or computer databank, despite appropriate protections, or 'bugs' an office, this would be a violation of privacy.

This situation is quite rare, but there are many everyday situations where confidentiality and/or privacy could be violated. The case considered in this chapter is related more to privacy than confidentiality, if the above distinction is strictly adhered to. However, in discussion, many practitioners use the term confidentiality to cover most situations relating to personal details. The following example indicates the differences between the two terms in a midwifery situation:

Midwife A conducts a booking interview and the woman explains that she has previously had a termination of pregnancy (TOP) but that her partner does not know.

1. If midwife A discloses this information to the partner, by intention or accident, she is guilty of a violation of confidentiality.

2. If midwife B, perhaps at a later clinic or during labour, discloses the information that she has read in the notes, she is also guilty of violating confidentiality.

3. If midwife B were to leave the delivery room, having closed the case notes, and the partner opens them and reads part or all of the contents, perhaps out of passing interest rather than malice, he is guilty of a violation of privacy.

4. If a situation occurred where the woman authorised the disclosure of information to her partner, the midwife is not guilty of any violation or infringement although, in effect, there is a loss of both confidentiality and privacy.

Purtilo (1993) indicates that confidentially and privacy can be linked, but are also separate issues. However, she states that maintaining confidentiality relates to 'harmful, shameful or embarrassing' information (p. 97). This terminology seems a little extreme. Who is to judge what any one woman might find harmful or embarrassing? If the healthcare professional concerned judges according to their own opinion, they may fall short of the standards that the woman would judge by.

With regard to client's/patient's records, there are two acts with which readers should be familiar. The first is the *Data Protection Act 1998*. This covers computer-held records and therefore affects most hospitals in the UK; clients can make application to view recorded information regarding themselves. The second is the *Access to Health Records Act 1990*, which came into force on 1 November 1991; adult clients are entitled to apply for access to any written records made after this date. If the client is a minor, then the usual situation regarding competence applies (see Ch. 7 on Autonomy and Consent). There are others who may be authorised to access a person's records but this, and the exemptions that may apply, will not be discussed here. If clients wish to access written records made before this date, they must make formal application, but they may be refused.

In situations 1 and 2 in the above example, the employing authority could also be accountable for the violations in accountability by vicarious liability, as they hold a degree of responsibility for the actions of staff in their employ (Mason & McCall Smith 1994).

FOR WHOM IS CONFIDENTIALITY/PRIVACY IMPORTANT?

It is not difficult to remember that confidentiality should be maintained for all the women in our care. However, we must realise that relatives also choose to confide in us. The author has had a number of experiences where the health of the woman has been poor, with severe pre-eclampsia in repeated pregnancies, moderate to severe renal disease or repeated puerperal psychosis, where sterilisation has been advised. In these particular cases it had been suggested that perhaps the partner could consider vasectomy rather than subject the woman to tubal ligation. In some of these cases the men confided that the partnerships were insecure and therefore future partnerships had to be considered. The consequences of violating such confidences, from the viewpoint of the families concerned, would be devastating and, as professionals, we must not help to create such an outcome.

Another group to be considered are colleagues, at all levels. Apart from personal confidences that friends and colleagues may confide or exchange, there are occasions where it is possible to observe incidents or overhear conversations. This could involve a colleague being counselled for an error or oversight, or a problem occurring during a delivery. It would be a violation of privacy to disclose this knowledge to another colleague and, even if this was in support of the one with a problem, it would still be an infringement.

The situation would be different, of course, if an incident was observed or overheard involving the probable act of misconduct of a member of staff; for instance, if there were apparent abuse of a woman or her baby (see Ch. 6 on Accountability), or an incident involving the administration of drugs, or evidence of drug or alcohol abuse by a member of staff. In any such situation, the observer should report the incident to her manager or Supervisor of Midwives. The privacy of a member of staff cannot be considered above the welfare of the women and their babies in our care (UKCC 1992, clause 13). The same would be the case with concerns regarding poor standards of care generally; this too should be reported to the manager or Supervisor of Midwives and not to an outside agency, as this could be deemed a violation of the service's confidentiality and therefore a breach of contract. The principles of clinical governance would expect all staff to alert proper authorities with regard to any elements of poor quality of care.

WHEN DO HEALTHCARE WORKERS NEED TO CONSIDER CONFIDENTIALITY/PRIVACY WITH REGARD TO INFORMATION?

There are many situations where care is required in the workplace. A woman's case notes, in whatever form, are obviously an area of concern, considering the amount and type of information recorded; it is important not to leave them available to onlookers or to allow other unauthorised access. This is an area where most midwives are probably very careful.

The 'report' conducted at a shift change, however, is not always considered with such concern. In some cases it occurs in a fairly public area of the ward or department, but even when greater privacy is sought it must be remembered that loud voices can travel through walls and down corridors. It is therefore possible for the woman being discussed, or any other woman or visitor, to overhear what is being said. Also, as stated previously, it could be that unnecessary information is given to staff who do not require it. The fact of a woman overhearing her own report is not particularly important in itself if she has been fully included in her own care. Problems arise when she feels that other women could hear personal details about her, or when staff have been unprofessional by making unpleasant subjective comments about her.

The telephone was a wonderful invention (generally speaking), but to staff on a busy ward or delivery suite it can be the bane of their lives. It can also be a tool for breaching confidentiality, however innocently. It is very tempting automatically to answer questions over the telephone, rather than asking the woman what she would like said. For instance, it is a regular occurrence to have people asking whether their friend or relative 'has had her baby yet and, if so, what did she have?'. It also seems to be a frequent occurrence that the caller is not the sister or mother-in-law that she claims to be, but a friend or neighbour. Midwives report that Christmas and New Year can create problems with the media: reporters from local press and television contact hospitals to determine whatever details they can regarding babies born on these occasions. Perhaps the worst of all is the estranged partner who, not admitting to the estrangement, asks: 'Can you tell me whether my wife/girlfriend has been admitted please? I have been trying to ring her from work, with no reply, and I am getting quite worried because she said she was not going out.' In all these situations it is so easy to answer, almost automatically, without really thinking of the consequences, especially during a very busy shift.

Meal breaks can be times when staff can be guilty of discussing many aspects of their work, including the interesting or difficult woman they were dealing with just before their break. This is not only failing to uphold the 'need to know' principle, but the conversation could be overheard by the woman's relative or neighbour, sitting at another table, who also works at the hospital; also, some hospitals have visitors sharing the same facilities as the staff.

Applying theory to practice is an essential part of the education of students. There is really no better way than for them to discuss actual cases that they have been involved in, especially if they are particularly elated or distressed by the case. However well the anonymity rule is observed, it is almost certain that another student will recognise the case from the delivery suite, clinic or neonatal unit. The author feels that students must have the benefit of such discussions, with the relief that often follows the discovery that someone else has also experienced such a situation. In order to do this, a room, possibly a classroom, should be designated a 'safe area' where discussions can take place freely, but where the rule is that discussion finishes within that room, with none of the information being discussed outside. Where assignment work is concerned, anonymity must always be observed; this is far easier because the work is prepared over a period of time, with time to think and plan properly, unlike the spontaneity experienced within a verbal discussion.

At the end of a working day or night it is hoped that the majority of staff go home to caring parents, partners, families or friends – people who are interested in what kind of day/night they have had. Possibly they have travelled home with colleagues on public transport, and perhaps they intend to go out for a meal with friends who find it fascinating to listen to tales of midwifery encounters. In all these situations it would be easy to relax and forget about confidentiality. To a great extent this is reasonable: midwives and other members of staff are not expected to be silent about their work; all that is required is that they maintain the confidentiality and privacy of the women/families in their care.

APPLYING THE THEORIES

Utilitarian views

With regard to Helen, the cost–benefit analysis would obviously suggest that she should be told about the error. Whether Anna should disregard the consultant's decision is the next problem. If Anna goes ahead and tells Helen, she might incur the wrath of Mr Fisch. On the other hand, if she waits until the registrar arrives, Helen could be further harmed by her continued anxieties; she might even contact her partner and create greater problems. Anna and Carmel would also find it very difficult to care for Helen adequately in the meantime. In balancing the consequences of her possible actions, the act-utilitarian would support Anna in correcting the error immediately; Helen would have to be told at some point and nothing good would be gained by waiting.

A rule-utilitarian would possibly make the same decision, probably following a rule that suggests it is never right to create suffering if no good comes from it.

With regard to Susan, an act-utilitarian may well consider that what she does not know probably will not harm her. Telling her would achieve no extra positive results other than the professionals knowing that they have been honest, whereas it could achieve negative results for Susan, the consultant and the hospital. Truth-telling is not an absolute principle or value to an act-utilitarian. To a rule-utilitarian this principle may be of more importance, considering that it is generally better for people to be truthful. However, they would still need to achieve greater benefit than harm and, unless asked directly by Susan (which could happen if she was indeed a client in the same bay and heard it all), the decision would probably be to keep quiet.

Deontological views

A Kantian would consider that one ought to be honest and face up to mistakes honourably; in general it would be considered immoral to hide mistakes or not tell the truth. Also, to uphold the principle of autonomy, clients should be kept informed. Therefore, the decision would probably be to tell both women what had occurred. Although it would be expected that Helen be told as soon as possible, a Kantian would probably expect that Mr Fisch should also come to apologise for the harm caused.

A traditionalist would probably follow the same action as a Kantian, from the honesty and honour point of view.

A pluralist would consider the prima-facie duties, in the order that seemed suitable to the case. Beneficence, non-maleficence, fidelity and justice would certainly feature highly. In Helen's case, there can be no doubt that a pluralist would want her to be told as soon as possible. In Susan's case, however, there could be some conflict between the principles. The duty of fidelity, where it would be considered that honesty would be part of the trusting relationship, might conflict with doing good and – more importantly – avoiding harm. It could depend on the individual and the order of importance in which they placed the principles, but the chances are that concern regarding the creation of harm would encourage him or her to say nothing.

REFERENCES

Anderson J 1996 Security in clinical information systems. British Medical Association, London

Beauchamp T L, Childress J F 1994 Principles of biomedical ethics, 4th edn. Oxford University Press, Oxford

Darley B, Griew A, McLoughlin K, Williams J 1994 How to keep a clinical confidence. HMSO, London

General Medical Council 1993 Professional conduct and discipline: fitness to practice. GMC, London

Lyndsay P 1997 Conditions and complications of pregnancy and labour. In: Sweet B (ed) Mayes' midwifery. A textbook for midwives, 12th edn. Baillière Tindall, London, p. 603

Mason J K, McCall Smith R A (1994) Law and medical ethics, 4th edn. Butterworths, London

Purtilo R 1993 Ethical dimensions in the health professions, 2nd edn. W B Saunders, Philadelphia, Pennsylvania, p. 93

Robinson J 1996 Confidentiality and the midwife. British Journal of Midwifery 4(12):666–667

Simpson C 1997 The newborn baby. In: Sweet B (ed) Mayes' midwifery. A textbook for midwives, 12th edn. Baillière Tindall, London, p. 896

UKCC 1992 Code of professional conduct for the nurse, midwife and health visitor. UKCC, London

UKCC 1996 Guidelines for professional practice. UKCC, London

SUGGESTED ADDITIONAL READING

Aziz B 1998 Confidential matters. Nursing Management 4(9):10–11

David T J, Wynne J, Kessel A S, Brazier M 1998 Child sexual abuse: when a doctor's duty to report abuse conflicts with a duty of confidentiality to the victim. British Medical Journal 316:55–57

Public Interest Disclosure Act 1998 HMSO, London

Tschudin V (ed) 1995 Ethics. The patient's charter. Scutari, Harrow

Wadham J, Mountfield H 1999 Blackstone's guide to the Human Rights Act 1998. Blackstone, London

6

Accountability

Michelle was a junior pre-registration student midwife who was undertaking a midwifery degree, having worked as a registered general nurse (RGN) in a local accident and emergency unit for two years. On the day in question, she and her named assessor, Edwina, were caring for a woman in established labour. The two professional women had a good working relationship, although Michelle was concerned that Edwina's manner with some of the clients was somewhat unorthodox.

The client on this occasion was an unaccompanied 24-year-old Muslim woman, Amal, having her first baby. She spoke very little English, but Michelle felt that her understanding was quite good and her spoken English was probably restricted more by lack of confidence than by lack of knowledge or ability. An interpreter had visited before Michelle and Edwina had taken over Amal's care and she had offered to come back as needed. As labour progressed Amal became distressed and what little English she had got seemed to disappear. As Amal became more disturbed, Edwina's already brusque manner worsened. Michelle suggested recalling the interpreter but Edwina said that it would not be necessary as Amal was nearing the second stage of labour.

Michelle tried to comfort Amal by touch and eye contact but, as Edwina had become verbally abusive, Amal became more frightened and the situation was getting out of hand. The level of noise in the room was rising, with Amal crying hysterically and Edwina shouting abusively at her and berating her for not speaking English. On two occasions different midwives, Barbara and Lucy, came into the room to see what the commotion was about. On each occasion Edwina stated that the client was out of control and she was dealing with it. Both midwives had asked Michelle if she was alright and, on both occasions, she had tried to indicate by non-verbal means that she was concerned about Edwina's behaviour. Lucy had shrugged her shoulders and shaken her head as if to indicate that there was nothing she could do. During the second stage of labour Amal remained distressed and frightened. On one occasion, when she straightened one leg while pushing instead of keeping the knee flexed, Edwina slapped her hard across the thigh. Michelle was stunned and Amal cried even more.

After the delivery, Michelle left the room on the pretext of collecting some clean linen; she was emotionally bruised by her experience. As she passed the staff station she heard midwives discussing Edwina's abusive manner with clients on this and other occasions. They suddenly went quiet when they realised Michelle was nearby. Barbara asked if she was alright, then told her not to worry as Edwina was often like that.

After two troubled days off duty, Michelle reported the incident to the labour ward manager. She was surprised to find that no-one else had reported it.

QUESTIONS FOR CONSIDERATION BY THE READER

1. Was Michelle right to report the incident?
2. Could Barbara or Lucy have done anything to help?
3. Does any responsibility rest with the other midwives on duty at that time?
4. What are the possible outcomes for Edwina if this incident is reported?

Issues that are not discussed here but which readers may wish to pursue include: culture, language and discrimination.

QUESTION 1: WAS MICHELLE RIGHT TO REPORT THE INCIDENT?

Although students cannot be held to account in accordance with the *Code of Professional Conduct* (UKCC 1992), they are advised to work towards it and, to this end, would be provided with a copy of the document. Students should, therefore, be familiar with the 16 clauses of the code, particularly clause 11 in this case, which directs the practitioner to report circumstances that could create harm.

Michelle was a registered nurse before taking up her place in midwifery education. It could be argued that she was using some of her nursing knowledge, skills and experience on a daily basis – in her general care and observations of a client – in the clinical settings. She should, therefore, know what is and is not acceptable behaviour, and would be expected to report such deviations from professional practice. Some people would suggest that, although the UKCC has stated: 'As a pre-registration student, you are never professionally accountable in the way that you will be after you come to register' (UKCC 1998a, p. 4), this should apply to situations that are midwifery specific and not of a general nature. A student on a shortened midwifery course has pre-registration status only for midwifery, not for all health care. Although the labour ward setting is midwifery specific, abusive behaviour towards a client is general, and a RGN would know that this is unacceptable behaviour, whereas a pre-registration student with no nursing background might presume only that it was unacceptable. It could also be argued, then, that failure of this student to report the situation could be deemed to be misconduct, whereas it would not be so for a pre-registration midwifery student on a long programme.

A similar view could be taken with regard to upholding the ethical codes inherent in the *Guidelines for Professional Practice* (UKCC 1996). This document indicates, among other points, the requirement for the practitioner to be the client's advocate (pp. 13–14) and the need to report inappropriate behaviour of a colleague (pp. 21–22). According to Bartter (1996, p. 222):

> *An advocate is a noble being, a courageous, honest individual who has good judgement and is sincere and tenacious to her task.*

With this definition, it is understandable that the professional body should require its practitioners to be such people.

Regardless of professional status, Michelle, as a fellow human being, should be concerned regarding Amal's treatment. Not only is her treatment lacking in beneficence, it is positively maleficent, which means that Edwina is in breach of at least two ethical principles. Members of the public rightly expect to be treated with care and compassion by all healthcare workers, particularly when they are most vulnerable, such as in labour. In order to protect future clients, therefore, she was right to report the incident.

QUESTION 2: COULD BARBARA OR LUCY HAVE DONE ANYTHING TO HELP?

Both midwives had entered the room, at different times, because of the noise. They must have heard Edwina shouting as well as Amal's hysterical crying. However, it might not have been possible to determine whether Edwina was raising her voice to be heard above Amal's hysteria, or actually shouting at her. Having entered the room, they would have had a better overall view of the situation. According to Michelle's description of events, it would appear that the midwives should have been able to sense the animosity and tension. They should have been able to see that Amal was frightened, although they might have assumed that it was due to fear of pain and delivery. Both midwives had asked Michelle if she was alright, which suggests that the atmosphere was threatening, and she had tried, by non-verbal means, to convey her concerns.

They could have considered Michelle's obvious concerns to be related to caring for a client who was out of control. If this were the case, it would seem more likely that they would have offered to relieve her for a short time, or at least offered her some support. In the event, both midwives left the room, effectively leaving both the client and the student unsupported in a hostile atmosphere. In fact, Lucy's body language suggested that she was well aware of what was happening but was unable or unwilling to do anything to help. She is just as accountable for her actions or omissions at this point as Edwina is for hers.

In truth, nobody is completely powerless in such a position; rather, they wish to avoid the inevitable discomfort brought about by confrontation. Both Barbara and Lucy, as qualified midwives of whatever grade, could have offered to relieve the midwife for a coffee break, thus breaking the tension and giving the opportunity for everyone to calm down. If the offer had been refused, or if they really felt unable to make the suggestion, then they should have reported the situation to the shift leader, assuming that this was not Edwina. The shift leader could have requested that Edwina step outside the room in order to speak to her, while sending in another midwife, or she could have relieved Edwina herself and dealt with the matter later. This would have created a break in continuity of carer; however, this concept is intended to promote emotional and physical well-being for the client and, in this case, neither was being achieved by continuity of this carer. If Edwina was the shift leader, then Barbara or Lucy should have contacted the manager on call, or the bleep-holder. Even if this person was not a midwife, she would have the authority to remove Edwina from the situation and initially counsel her as to her conduct, perhaps even suspending her from duty.

Another person who could be contacted is a Supervisor of Midwives. She has a responsibility for promoting and maintaining safety for the mother and baby and, while Edwina may have been able to deliver the mother of her baby safely, or supervise Michelle's delivery, Amal's personal safety proved to be in jeopardy. The Supervisor is also responsible for protecting and supporting the midwives. She could have counselled Edwina to ascertain the reason for her behaviour, then provided appropriate support and guidance.

Barbara and Lucy took no positive action at the time or subsequently. In addition, they may or may not have been the instigators of the discussion that was taking place at the staff station when Michelle walked past. As stated earlier, these qualified midwives must abide by the *Code of Professional Conduct* (UKCC 1992, clause 11), which requires midwives to:

> *Report to an appropriate person or authority, having regard to the physical, psychological and social effects on patients and clients, any circumstances in the environment of care which could jeopardise standards of practice.*

QUESTION 3: DOES ANY RESPONSIBILITY REST WITH THE OTHER MIDWIVES ON DUTY AT THAT TIME?

From the discussion taking place at the staff station, it is apparent that Edwina had a reputation for abusive conduct. It has to be assumed that this behaviour had never been reported officially or dealt with effectively for it to be occurring on this occasion. It is understandable that a midwife's first reaction to the inappropriate behaviour of another midwife is to ignore it and hope that it will pass. We are socialised from early in our lives that 'telling tales' is not good behaviour. However, a midwife's behaviour in dealing with clients or relatives is of greater importance than the minor misdemeanours of a child. Reflection by the midwives might have made them consider Edwina's privacy, which might have led them to believe that they could not report the incident. However, this would suggest that the midwife's privacy was of greater importance than the client's right to proper non-abusive care and attention.

The document *Guidelines for Professional Practice* (UKCC 1996) provides an expansion or explanation of the *Code of Professional Conduct* (UKCC 1992). It states that clauses 1–4 are to ensure that practitioners put the interests of their clients before those of themselves or their colleagues. Barbara and Lucy, although not present for the slap on the thigh, were aware of the verbal assault on Amal; therefore, they were duty bound, according to the Code, to report the incident to the manager on duty. In doing so, not only would they be observing their professional duty, they would be protected by the *Public Interest Disclosure Act 1998 (sections 43B(1) & 43C(1))*.

It is often said that midwives do not stand together, as is the case with their medical colleagues; rather, they will be the first to criticise the actions or omissions of other midwives. Although this may be true, as observed by Michelle as she passed the staff station, they tend to gossip amongst themselves rather than reporting to someone in authority. Perhaps they believe that this acknowledges rather than ignores the fact that the behaviour is unacceptable, without being so disloyal to the colleague as to report them officially. Where midwives comment on medical unity, is their view that we should emulate such colleagues? – colleagues who have been encouraged by their professional body, the General Medical Council, 'not to initiate action against colleagues, or to break the culture of mutual cover-up' and instructed that 'disparaging the services of a fellow practitioner is an offence' (Palmer 1995, p. 9).

This behaviour is greatly criticised by midwives when they believe that a doctor's actions or omissions have caused harm to a client, or have disparaged a midwife – and rightly so. No healthcare professional should be able to abuse his or her privileged position, and fellow professionals should be prepared to highlight abuse and poor practice. If they are not prepared to do this, 'do they deserve the right to police their own professional standards?' (Jones 1996, p. 297). Unfortunately, there appear to be sufficient cases of abuse of privilege, of various kinds, that the UKCC (1999, p. 4) has produced a guidance document for practitioners which states:

> *Zero tolerance of abuse is the only philosophy consistent with protecting the public.*

QUESTION 4: WHAT ARE THE POSSIBLE OUTCOMES FOR EDWINA OF THIS INCIDENT BEING REPORTED?

If this incident had been reported to the manager on duty at the time, Edwina would probably have been removed from the situation and replaced by another midwife. She may well be suspended from duty after an initial discussion with the manager, at least for the remainder of that shift. If it was a non-midwife manager, the situation would be explained to the midwife manager in the next handover.

As it was, the incident was reported to the labour ward manager three days later. The manager could take one of two courses of action: she could inform the relevant Supervisor of Midwives and request that a supervisory investigation be carried out, or she could notify the Supervisor, in order to provide professional support for Edwina, and conduct a management investigation herself. Deciding to pacify the student while taking no further action is not an option. The manager is accountable for her practice also, and this includes ensuring that the business of the Trust is carried out in a safe and acceptable manner. As the allegations involve possible gross misconduct rather than an error of clinical judgement, it is likely that both the manager and Supervisor would carry out investigations; these may be separate, or the two people could conduct a single investigation involving both the employment and professional pathways.

From the management point of view, it is probable that Edwina would be suspended from duty, following an initial opportunity for the midwife to explain her actions. Therefore, she will be unable to return to her work in that unit until the investigation and relevant meetings have been completed. This action serves two purposes. First, it allows the midwife some time away from the unit to reflect on her situation and the events as they occurred; because of any underlying problems, or the effect of the incident itself, Edwina may feel unable to work at this time anyway. Second, it allows for a smoother investigation as the individuals involved might feel more comfortable making statements and being interviewed when the subject of the investigation is not around to observe or, in some cases, even intimidate them.

As soon as possible after the incident, Edwina would be asked for her account of the events described. She would be advised to seek assistance from her Supervisor and a professional representative, such as a steward for the Royal College of Midwives, when writing her statement of events. Managers and Supervisors can request advice and assistance from the human resources department to ensure that they abide by relevant rules (English National Board 1997).

Once the manager has gathered statements from Michelle, Edwina, Barbara and Lucy, she may choose to approach the client for her view of the incident, unless she has already received a complaint. On completion of the investigation, the manager will determine what course of action is required. In view of the nature of the complaint, if the investigation indicates a case to be answered, a disciplinary hearing will be arranged as soon as possible. If the allegation of misconduct is proved, then Edwina's disciplinary history and any pleas of mitigation will be taken into account when determining the action to be taken. Her honesty and remorse, if she admitted behaving inappropriately, will also be taken into account. Disciplinary action can take the form of verbal or written warnings, or dismissal. Dismissal can be the action determined in one of two ways. The first way is by accumulation of incidents, whereby the individual has previously reached the final warning stage of the process and is found to be in breach of contract while the final warning is still current. The second way is that the employee is found to have committed gross misconduct which allows the bypassing of warnings. If Edwina does not have any current warnings on file, if she has mitigating circumstances and is honest and remorseful, she would probably receive a written warning to remain on file for one or two years. If, however, she has warnings on file or she denies what the investigation has proved and is therefore remorseless, she is more likely to be dismissed. She can appeal against any disciplinary action which she deems unfair, within set time limits, including an appeal to an industrial tribunal for unfair dismissal.

The supervisory pathway of the investigation would be seeking to maintain the safety of mothers and babies as the first priority, followed by the provision of support for the midwife. While nobody would wish to prejudge Edwina's conduct before a full investigation, if initial investigation suggests that she is unsafe, or could cause harm to another mother or baby, the Supervisor of Midwives should notify the local supervising authority (LSA). The responsible officer for the LSA would determine whether Edwina should be suspended from practice. If Edwina receives a letter to this effect from the LSA, she will not be able to practice as a midwife within the area covered by that LSA until a UKCC investigation has been conducted. She could, however, work as a nurse if she has the relevant UKCC registration, or she could work as a midwife in another area covered by a different LSA. If the responsible officer considers that Edwina is a serious threat to mothers or babies and would be likely to be removed from the professional register following full investigation, she could request the UKCC to issue an interim suspension from the register, while awaiting full details of the case. This would usually prevent Edwina from practising under any UKCC registration anywhere in the UK (ENB 1997).

Assuming that such drastic measures are not taken, the Supervisor would ensure that professional support is provided which will help Edwina to determine her professional needs. These needs may involve development of specific knowledge, skills or attitudes; they may also involve being moved from the labour ward, or provision of a period of supervised practice. If the named Supervisor is undertaking the investigation, another Supervisor will provide the support.

FURTHER DISCUSSION

If a group of students or qualified midwives is asked for a definition of accountability, in the author's experience, it is usual to hear 'responsibility for one's actions', which of course is quite right. It is possible, however, that the importance of this is still not fully appreciated. In dictionaries, of various types and dates, accountability generally equates to 'responsibility'; however, use of a thesaurus may create a deeper perspective. The author would encourage readers to consider the term to include duty and liability, thus 'being accountable' would equate to being 'responsible' and 'answerable'.

As midwives, we are accountable for ethical practice, which at least includes practising justly, beneficently, non-maleficently and with truthfulness. If we fail in upholding these principles, then we are answerable in civil law.

For whom and what are midwives accountable?

It is obvious that the women and their babies feature high on the list, with midwives being responsible for their safety and general well-being, including educating the women into safe care of their babies. There is also responsibility for the family as a whole; midwives are ideally placed to tackle aspects of health promotion with or for the whole family. It is also their duty to observe for, and assist with, the healthy integration of the baby into the family, thus helping to prevent some of the physical and mental traumas that can occur if integration is delayed, particularly for the mother and baby. The government report *Making a Difference* (Department of Health 1999) states quite clearly that the midwife's role could be expanded to include all aspects of women's health. While this is a logical and welcome move forward, it continues to expand the responsibility of the midwife.

In some respects, all midwives are accountable for their colleagues, of all grades, in maintaining safe and harmonious team-work. Observance of general health and safety principles are essential, such as giving proper attention to the disposal of sharp objects and care when dealing with body fluids. As for harmony, if this is lacking then it can create a stressful working atmosphere, which may affect not only the health and well-being of the staff, but possibly also the care received by the clients, and certainly would create a bad image to clients and their visitors.

The 'what' in the question generally relates to equipment. Technological equipment is expensive and often temperamental through over-use; it should be handled with care. It should be remembered that the appropriate technicians are the only people who are approved to correct the faults (many of which could be prevented by responsible handling) – not a midwife who is handy with a screwdriver or a blade from her scissors! Machinery is often used and abused by many – even the husbands at times – therefore the midwife can be held responsible only for any specific damage or negligence caused by her.

The above points are slightly different from what we usually consider to be actual accountability; however, the midwife is accountable for any acts and omissions pertaining to these areas. It therefore seems logical to include them here.

Accountability is one of the areas that is highlighted in discussions regarding the difference between midwifery and nursing. In looking through the above areas of responsibility, the reader could be forgiven for considering that there is no difference in accountability; in fact, the next three areas are those that create part of the difference.

Under the *Congenital Disabilities (Civil Liability) Act 1976*, a midwife can be held accountable for any act or omission committed by her which has resulted in damage to the fetus or baby. Action can be taken on behalf of the child, up to the age of 18 years; once (s)he reaches 18, the action must be taken by the person her/himself up to the age of 21 years. This extra three years comes from the statutory right that any adult has, under the *Limitations Act 1980*, to bring a claim within three years of knowledge of the possible cause of the problem. If the person, once adult, is considered mentally incompetent, then an advocate can represent her/him and the time does not end after three years: it is indefinite. It can take four years for the case to reach the courts; therefore, a midwife could be in the position of having to interpret her records up to 25 years after the event. This in itself indicates the need for full and accurate record-keeping, and guidance is given by the UKCC (1998b). The effects of the *Congenital Disabilities (Civil Liability) Act 1976* were expected to relate to cases occurring after the Act came into force; however, the Court of Appeal ruled that two claimants, whose injuries had occurred before the Act, could continue with their claim under common law (Dyer 1992).

Midwives are permitted to carry and prescribe certain drugs. Their exemption from the *Misuse of Drugs Act 1971* permits them to carry out specific functions with particular drugs, but only in accordance with their sphere of practice. They cannot, for instance, give intramuscular pethidine to a client's husband who is in severe pain from renal colic. Although there is the facility for midwives to carry various drugs, they do not necessarily do so. They must abide by local policies regarding the actual drugs and quantities carried. In doctor-led units, midwives would generally follow similar rules to nurses, in accordance with individual medication sheets or by following protocols (Department of Health 1998). In the community, practice is essentially different but in current practice, for reasons of safety, midwives rarely carry prescription-only medicines (POMs), such as pethidine, and women who intend to labour and deliver at home often obtain the required drugs by prescription.

Since 1994, some nurses have been able to supply and administer certain POMs. This was enabled by the *Medicinal Products: Prescription by Nurses etc. Act 1992* (amended), which permits registered district nurses, health visitors and some nurses with specialist practice qualifications to prescribe from a *Nurse Prescribers' Formulary*. These practitioners must be in primary care, they must have undergone appropriate training, be identified by the UKCC and must be authorised by their employers to prescribe (Courtenay & Butler 1999). In these cases this particular difference between nurses and midwives no longer exists; however, by far the majority of registered nurses are not able to prescribe and administer without prescriptions or protocols.

There is also specific accountability with regard to notification and registration of births and deaths. It is usually the midwife who notifies the birth that she has attended, within 36 hours, and the mother and/or father who register(s) the baby within 42 days of the birth. If the parents neglect to register the baby, then it is the duty of the midwife. This does not mean that she needs to seek them out at 41 days after delivery; rather, she would be contacted by the Registrar's office. The personnel in this office would know to await the registration, as the birth had already been notified. As for deaths, it would normally be the responsibility of the doctor who certified the mother, stillborn baby or neonate dead who would complete the death or stillbirth certificate and issue it to the family for them to register the death. If a registered medical practitioner is not available for some reason, the duty falls to the midwife present at the delivery;

so too does the duty to register the death, if the family fail to do this (UKCC 1998a).

To whom are midwives accountable?

First, the midwife is accountable to the family, of which the mother is an integral member. As stated earlier, if the midwife fails to observe ethical practice she can face the consequences in civil law. A breach in her duties to mother or baby, resulting in either of them suffering harm, could cause them to sue her in the civil courts; one such law suit would be for negligence. For the woman, or her legal adviser(s), to prove negligence against a midwife it would be necessary to prove, on the balance of probabilities, that the midwife:

◆ had a duty of care to the woman
◆ that she breached her duty of care
◆ that the harm in question was caused by the breach of duty and nothing else.

Before analysing the case under discussion, it is necessary to indicate the legal definition of the *'duty of care'.* The definition was determined in 1932 by Lord Atkin, in the case of Donoghue v Stevenson. He stated:

> *You must take reasonable care to avoid acts and omissions which you can reasonably foresee would be likely to injure your neighbour. ... persons who are so closely and directly affected by my act that I ought to have them in contemplation as being so affected when I am directing my mind to the acts and omissions which are called in question. (UKCC 1996, p. 10).*

The ethical underpinning of this definition obviously involves the principles and duties of beneficence and non-maleficence. It also involves consequentialism, as it requires individuals to use reasonable foresight in determining courses of action.

In the case under discussion, it is obvious that Edwina had a duty of care for Amal (Montgomery 1997). She was the named midwife allocated for that episode of care and her acts and omissions would definitely have some impact on Amal. The next consideration is whether she breached her duty of care. This would be judged according to the Bolam test, which was derived from the case of

Bolam v Friern Hospital Management Committee (1957) and applied here to a midwifery situation:

> ...*the standard of the ordinary skilled [midwife] exercising and professing to have that special skill. A [midwife] need not possess the highest expert skill ... it is sufficient that [she] exercises the skill of an ordinary competent [midwife] exercising that particular art.* (Dimond 1994, p. 28)

It is unlikely that any practising midwife would suggest that verbal and physical abuse formed part of the skill of an ordinary competent midwife. To do so would suggest that ordinary midwifery practice lacked care and observance of basic human rights and dignity, that it failed to observe the basic principles and duties of ethical practice. Edwina would be deemed to have breached her duty of care; her standard of care for Amal was so poor that no other reasonably competent midwife would have given that care (Symon 1998).

Causation is the last and most difficult aspect to prove. In part it would depend on what Amal claimed the harm to be and whether she could prove it. She could claim fear and actual trespass to her person, which could be attested to by Michelle. She could also claim that her potential satisfaction with her labour had been destroyed by Edwina's behaviour. However, it could not be proved that the natural pain of labour was not to blame and perhaps she would not have felt satisfied with the experience in any case. Discussion with psychiatrists and psychiatric nurses suggests that there is a definite increase in diagnosed cases of post-traumatic stress disorder in postnatal women who experienced emotionally or physically traumatic labours or deliveries. It is possible that a case such as the one outlined could result in such a disorder and causation might be proved. According to Kidner (1992), people cannot be protected totally against risks and can be compensated only where unreasonable activity has caused damage. He indicates that there are two opposing questions to ask. In this case, did the midwife create unreasonable risk? And what level of safety was Amal entitled to expect? A reasonable midwife would consider that Amal was entitled to expect safety from abuse and that Edwina not only created unreasonable risk, but actual harm.

Edwina would appear to be the culprit in this situation; she would be expected to give evidence and would undoubtedly feel the pressure of the allegations. However, the Trust bears vicarious liability for its employees, while working within the course of their employment, and would actually face the financial pressures of a successful claim in negligence.

The midwife is accountable to the UKCC for her conduct and it is for the Professional Conduct Committee of the council to determine whether she is guilty of conduct unworthy of a midwife, and therefore guilty of misconduct (Dimond 1994); such a verdict could result in the midwife being removed from the register (UKCC 1998a). As indicated earlier, the investigation and disciplinary process usually begins with the Supervisor of Midwives. The UKCC document *Guidelines for Professional Practice* (1996) seeks to assist practitioners in the important area of accountability. It is also expected by the Government that midwives fully understand their obligations to the clients in their care, and that they work within the framework of statutory regulation (Department of Health 1999).

Accountability to her employer is the next aspect to consider. A midwife is contracted to carry out the duties for which she is employed in accordance with the statutory rules and codes; also, she must adhere to the local policies within the employing authority. Any breach of duty to the woman and/or baby in her care could be considered to be a breach in contract, thus resulting in possible dismissal.

The last – but very important – person to be considered is the midwife herself. The author firmly believes that accountability to oneself should not be dismissed as unimportant in the face of other agents of accountability. Everyone makes mistakes, some more regrettable than others, but whether these mistakes are punished by another agency or not, the knowledge of that error will stay with that midwife forever – a fact she should keep in mind throughout her professional activities.

As the twentieth century progressed, so the face of midwifery changed. Although the principles behind accountability remained largely the same, the variety of activities in which a midwife might be involved blossomed. Currently, not all midwives are involved in all the new aspects, but they are obviously accountable for their part in any which they undertake. These activities include provision of contraceptive advice, preconception counselling, ultrasonographic scanning, perineal suturing, epidural top-ups, venepuncture, cannulation, and even forceps or vacuum delivery. With the advent of electronic fetal monitoring, midwives had to learn how to use the machinery and interpret the readings.

One of the most difficult areas faced by midwives is probably the observance of the penultimate activity, listed in the European Union *Midwives Directive 80/155/EEC* article 4, which states (UKCC 1998c, p. 26):

> ...*to carry out treatment prescribed by a doctor.*

This is particularly difficult when that doctor may only just be starting in obstetric experience. Obviously midwives are at liberty to discuss decisions made by such doctors, and can often offer advice, but a lot depends on the doctor's willingness to accept the advice and the midwife's manner in giving it. In many units, it would appear, junior doctors are considered 'junior' to the experienced midwives; in others, such doctors are not permitted to make decisions in the delivery suite – unless of a general medical nature.

The author would suggest that midwives should not find the above clause so difficult. There are many situations where the 'treatments prescribed' are concerned with high-risk cases or non-midwifery/obstetric matters, where it is the doctor's province. In the midwifery/obstetric field, if the midwife feels that she cannot carry out the doctor's wishes then she should not do so. She should explain why she feels unable to do so, inviting the doctor either to change the instruction or to conduct the procedure personally. Accountability cannot be transferred; if the midwife follows a course of action that leads to difficulty, it would be useless for her to stand up in court, or at the UKCC and state: 'The doctor told me to'. The doctor may well be guilty of an error of judgement, but an error no greater than that of the midwife who carried out what she knew to be an unsafe procedure, therefore failing in her duties of beneficence and non-maleficence.

APPLYING THE THEORIES

Utilitarian views

Utilitarians view the prospective consequences of an act in terms of good or benefit. In this case, Edwina's verbal and physical abuse of the client could be predicted to cause harm and distress rather than any good; therefore, it would be deemed to be a bad act and should not be undertaken. If the intended abuse was to shout in order to break through the hysteria, to enable the woman to regain control, then an act-utilitarian would probably accept the action, as this would create overall good. A rule-utilitarian, on the other hand, would question whether a general rule allowing midwives to shout at clients who have lost control would create more good. As it is unlikely that this would be the case, the rule-utilitarian would be against it.

With regard to Michelle's reporting of the incident, an act-utilitarian's cost–benefit analysis would consider that harm would befall Edwina, in the form of disciplinary action, on the cost side. However, benefit should be achieved hopefully by preventing her from causing harm to other women in the future. Reporting Edwina would, therefore, be a good act overall. A rule-utilitarian would also consider the cost–benefit analysis, but it would relate to having a general rule that requires that abusive midwives be reported. Again, for each midwife who is in this situation, there could be many women who would be saved from abusive behaviour; it would therefore be moral to have such a rule.

Deontological views

Kantians believe in treating people as ends in themselves and not as a means to someone else's ends, that is, not using or abusing them. Edwina did not treat Amal with such respect, rather she did abuse her. Kantian beliefs also include the principle of universalisation: would it be right to treat all labouring women in this way? Obviously, this would not be acceptable, so this action fails both tests and would be deemed immoral. As the act is immoral, it should not go unpunished; therefore, Michelle was right to report it – she was doing what she *ought* to do. The other midwives, in not reporting what they knew of the incident, could be seen to be failing in their moral duty to the woman.

Traditionalists would deem abusive behaviour to be unacceptable. They would also expect Edwina to be disciplined for her immoral behaviour; therefore, Michelle would be seen to have acted appropriately.

Pluralists would consider Edwina to have breached her duties of beneficence, non-maleficence and justice (and reparation if she does not make amends). This would definitely be immoral conduct. With regard to Michelle reporting the incident, the care of future clients would not be considered, only Michelle's duties to Amal and Edwina. The incident had already happened when she reported it, so she would not be creating any good for, or preventing any harm to, Amal. She could be seen to be obeying her duty of justice for Amal, with regard to fair play, but again it is after the event. In addition to her duties to Amal, Michelle has duties to Edwina, as another human being. The duty of fidelity suggests that she should be loyal to Edwina and say nothing that could cause her harm. Reporting the incident will undoubtedly equate to causing harm. Michelle would be caught in a dilemma, having conflicting duties to the two other women. The decision would probably be that Michelle would be right to report the incident, but only if she did it at the time, when there was time to change the emotional climate in order to benefit Amal and prevent some of the harm.

REFERENCES

Bartter K 1996 The midwife advocate. In: Frith L (ed) Ethics and midwifery. Butterworth–Heinemann, Oxford

Bolam v Friern Hospital Management Committee 1957 2 All E R 118

Courtenay M, Butler M 1999 Nurse prescribing. Principles and practice. Greenwich Medical Media, London

Department of Health 1998 Review of prescribing, supply and administration of medicines (Crown report). HMSO, London

Department of Health 1999 Making a difference. Strengthening the nursing, midwifery and health visiting contribution to health and healthcare. HMSO, London

Dimond B 1994 The legal aspects of midwifery. Books for Midwives Press, Hale, UK

Donoghue v Stevenson 1932 AC 562

Dyer C 1992 New ruling may fuel surge in birth damage cases. British Medical Journal 304(6832):937

English National Board 1997 Preparation of Supervisors of Midwives. Distance learning pack, module 4. ENB, London

Jones S R 1996 Client abuse and the personal cost of accountability. British Journal of Midwifery 4(6):295–297

Kidner R 1992 Casebook on torts, ch 5. Blackstone, London

Montgomery J 1997 Health care law. Oxford University Press, Oxford

Palmer A 1995 Now then, what seems to be the trouble? The Spectator 29 July:9–12

Symon A 1998 Litigation: the views of midwives and obstetricians. Hochland & Hochland, Hale, UK

UKCC 1992 Code of professional conduct for the nurse, midwife and health visitor. UKCC, London

UKCC 1996 Guidelines for professional practice. UKCC, London

UKCC 1998a A UKCC guide for students of nursing and midwifery. UKCC, London
UKCC 1998b Guidelines for records and record keeping. UKCC, London
UKCC 1998c Midwives rules and code of practice. UKCC, London
UKCC 1999 Practitioner–client relationships and the prevention of abuse. UKCC, London

SUGGESTED ADDITIONAL READING

General Medical Services Committee 1997 General practitioners and intrapartum care: interim guidance. BMA, London
Kennedy I 1988 Treat me right. Clarendon Press, Oxford
UKCC 1998 Complaints about professional conduct. UKCC, London

7

Autonomy and consent

Gary is a midwife in a community midwifery team which undertakes caseload practice. Most of his Sundays on duty include some home visits to undertake antenatal booking histories. Sometimes this is to enable both partners to be present, if the woman requests it, or to fit into the busy lives of working women. On this particular Sunday, Gary was undertaking such a visit to Caroline, a 32-year-old primiparous woman, and her partner Otto.

After some informal conversation to create a relaxed atmosphere, Gary started the more formal, but generally open, questioning required to gain as complete a picture of Caroline's past history and current state of health as possible. It appeared that Caroline had no adverse personal or family history: she was a fit and healthy woman who was 14 weeks into her first pregnancy. She and Otto were very pleased about the pregnancy; it was planned and there had been no delay in achieving conception. Both partners were journalists and Otto travelled a lot in the course of his international work. Caroline travelled less, being responsible for health-related articles for a women's magazine in the UK.

For the rest of the meeting, Gary let Caroline determine the order of issues discussed, although he was prepared to introduce essential issues if they were not raised by her. There was a long discussion about screening for fetal abnormality, about which Caroline was very well informed, having researched for an article on antenatal screening the previous year. Caroline and Otto were in favour of screening, although they were not sure what their reaction would be if faced with a high-risk result. Gary gave them the current information leaflet used in that area and an appointment for having the blood taken. They also discussed general health issues such as diet and exercise.

Caroline spoke as if it was automatic that she would deliver in the local hospital, but asked about the organisation of antenatal appointments. Gary asked whether Caroline wanted midwife-led care, explaining that this was client-centred and delivered mainly by midwives. He explained how the caseload team worked, with particular regard to continuity of care and carer where possible. Caroline stated that she would prefer more input from the team midwives than from doctors. Gary then proceeded to explain what was on offer for labour and delivery. The possibilities included hospital delivery, usually with a team midwife, with transfer home usually between six and 48 hours after delivery; this also included waterbirth, if the pool was vacant at the time. Another option was home delivery, including waterbirth if the client wished to hire the appropriate pool; but Gary pointed out that home delivery of any kind was not usually advised for first babies. Caroline asked about caesarean section as an option and Gary indicated that this was used only in complicated cases. Caroline stated that she had recently undertaken a literature search for an article on perineal trauma and, based on her findings, although she wanted midwifery care for everything else, she intended to request a caesarean section for delivery.

Gary decided not to pursue the discussion at that time, as he did not want to risk damaging the initial rapport that had been created. He suggested that she should discuss the issue with the consultant obstetrician, for whose clinic she would be sent an appointment.

QUESTIONS FOR CONSIDERATION BY THE READER

1. Should Gary have continued to discuss the issue of elective caesarean section?
2. Is the consultant obstetrician likely to concur with Caroline's wishes?
3. Should caesarean section be an option for any woman?

QUESTION 1: SHOULD GARY HAVE CONTINUED TO DISCUSS THE ISSUE OF ELECTIVE CAESAREAN SECTION?

Gary has shown his willingness to conduct client-led care. He has been prepared to provide information and the opportunity for open discussion around the choices open to Caroline. In short, he appears to have treated Caroline as an autonomous person. Why should his approach change when faced with a decision with which he might not agree?

Caroline has made her initial decision based on her interpretation of the literature search that she carried out for the magazine. She has shown rational, self-governed and self-controlled behaviour which indicates that she is an autonomous person (Beauchamp & Childress 1994). She is adult and apparently has not shown any obvious signs of psychiatric disorder; therefore, there was no reason to suggest that she be considered to have even a temporary loss of autonomy. If Gary was to continue with the discussion, he would need to outline the benefits and risks of caesarean section without bias. Caroline might become defensive, particularly if there was any suggestion of bias in the way Gary dealt with the issue, and this could cause antagonism in what appears to be the start of a good professional relationship. Antagonism would serve no purpose, especially as it will not be Gary's decision as to whether surgical intervention should be planned. This will be the consultant obstetrician's remit.

Gary has made a good start in developing effective communication with Caroline. He has started a partnership with her, indicated his ability to listen, and formed the basis of trust (UKCC 1996), which is an essential element in a professional relationship. Caroline has carefully selected the path that she wishes to follow, initially at least, during this major life experience. She will be looking to her midwife to assist her in the safe achievement of her plans. As she has not asked for his opinion, he is right to leave further discussion to the relevant consultant. The consultant will have to discuss the issue with Caroline and, as the gaining of consent for surgery is the remit of doctors, not midwives, determine how much information to give.

QUESTION 2: IS THE CONSULTANT OBSTETRICIAN LIKELY TO CONCUR WITH CAROLINE'S WISHES?

An unhelpful, but nevertheless reasonable, answer is probably that it would depend on the individual consultant. Some obstetricians, for whatever reasons – belief that caesarean section provides the least risk or no greater risk than vaginal delivery, or as defensive practice, or even to prevent midwifery taking over (Montgomery 1997) – have higher rates of caesarean section than others. All obstetricians will have emergency cases, although anecdotal evidence suggests that some will decide on surgical intervention much earlier than others. However, it is probably the rate of elective caesarean section that would give an indication as to their general views regarding the procedure.

Obstetricians appear to be divided on the issue. Those who believe that caesarean section holds few risks, particularly with modern anaesthesia, may well consider that it should feature in the menu of choices open to women. They may consider that women's preference, if based on full information and sound reason, should be upheld (Paterson-Brown, 1998). Some may even go so far as to believe that even 'foolish or irrational choices' should be upheld (Amu et al 1998), for that is the legal position with regard to a woman who refuses a caesarean section when it is advised (Dyer 1997). However, an obstetrician who still considers that the dangers of even elective surgical intervention are greater than those of a well observed labour and vaginal delivery will probably be reluctant to agree to this choice.

It is accepted that doctors have autonomy of practice, making their own decisions regarding their choice of management of cases. However, within the doctor's duty of care lies the duty to help the patient/client (beneficence), as well as the more stringent duty to do no harm (non-maleficence). The cost–benefit analysis of and between elective caesarean section and vaginal delivery should, therefore, be an essential exercise for the doctor concerned. The duty of care also includes the duty to inform the patient of significant risks. While there is no legal principle of informed consent in the UK, doctors and other health professionals could be accused of negligence if patients/clients considered that they were inadequately informed.

It would seem, therefore, that the obstetrician who will be faced with Caroline's request should inform her of the advantages and disadvantages of elective caesarean section, bearing in mind the fact that there may be no clinical need for the procedure. While the benefits regarding protection of Caroline's perineum in labour may be compelling, she would need to be informed that hormonal activity during pregnancy has an effect on the tone of the perineum, in which case she cannot be certain that she will regain full tone post-natally by avoiding vaginal delivery. The risks include the higher risk, albeit very small, of maternal death and possible neonatal morbidity, particularly with regard to lung function. Also, there will be some degree of post-surgical morbidity for the mother, which may create difficulties for her with regard to caring for her baby in the early days. In addition, there is the potential for adverse effects on a future pregnancy: reduced fertility and increased chance of conditions such as placenta praevia and accreta (Page 1999), as well as some other possible long-term effects (Amu et al 1998).

It would appear that a number of female obstetricians would opt for caesarean section (Al-Mufti et al 1997) but, as Page (1999) suggests, their views may be swayed by the fact that they are surrounded by complications and are skilled in surgical techniques, rather than normal vaginal delivery. Robinson (1998), also commenting on Al-Mufti et al's survey, suggested that, as most deliveries are undertaken by midwives, it would be interesting to know what they would choose.

Since the publication of the report *Changing Childbirth* (Department of Health 1993), client choice has been used and abused on a frequent basis. While most, but not all, midwives and doctors involved in childbirth experiences support the notion of women's choice, many have used it to avoid the restrictive policies and protocols within which they are supposed to work. Anecdotal evidence suggests that, where a midwife thinks that a certain course of action, contrary to the policy, is in the best interests of the woman, she will make appropriately worded suggestions to the woman. When the woman agrees with the midwife, the midwife writes something to the effect that the action or omission was according to the woman's wishes or request. It could be argued that this lacks a degree of veracity and is therefore unethical practice; however, if the midwife really believes that her actions were based on beneficence and non-maleficence, it could be deemed to be highly ethical.

Something similar was reported by Jean Robinson, as honorary research officer of the Association for Improvements in the Maternity Services (AIMS). She stated that one woman who had read her case notes discovered that the reason given for her surgical intervention was 'maternal choice' (Robinson 1998). The woman's version of events was that 'the obstetrician had strongly advised it and she had meekly agreed'. A second situation (Robinson 1999) involved a midwife seeing 'maternal request' as the reason for a woman's caesarean section, which she knew to be untrue, as she had been present at the consultation between the woman and her obstetrician.

An obstetrician could feel threatened by a request such as Caroline's. He or she could view it as a true dilemma where, whatever decision was taken, it would not be the perfect one. If the obstetrician agreed to undertake the caesarean section and a complication occurred, the woman could say that she had not been made sufficiently aware of the potential problem. She may even plead that the doctor should have refused her request given his or her knowledge of what was best. This would amount to a request for paternalism after the event. If the obstetrician refused to undertake the caesarean section and a problem occurred with the mother or fetus, again there could be a law suit.

Despite the dilemma, a decision has to be made and it should be made according to the clinical judgement of the doctor concerned. He has individual accountability and might find it difficult to justify his actions, if required to, based on a client's request rather than on sound clinical judgement (Dimond 1999).

QUESTION 3: SHOULD CAESAREAN SECTION BE AN OPTION FOR ANY WOMAN?

Autonomy is the principle at the heart of this debate. This principle (explained in Further discussion) requires the individual to be rational in their determination. If we believe in autonomy then we should believe in rational choice, but for many people, particularly most healthcare professionals, it would not seem rational for a woman to request a caesarean section where there is no known or perceived problem. However, a woman may have various reasons for such a request. She may have had a previous experience of childbirth which she viewed as particularly traumatic. Perhaps a history of childhood sexual abuse, or rape in any of a number of situations, could create a fear of vaginal delivery. Some women may be afraid that pain relief in labour will be inadequate, whereas post-operative pain relief may be anticipated as being better, or they may be afraid of losing control.

In other situations the reason may be that women need to be able to plan, as much is as possible, for this life event to fit into their lives; or it may be that they really do perceive caesarean section as a greater guarantee of achieving a perfect outcome of their pregnancy. Some obstetricians would agree with this view.

If it is considered suitable for a woman to request a caesarean section for non-clinical reasons then, within the realms of justice, we should be offering it in our menu of options; otherwise we could be seen to be discriminating against those who do not ask for themselves. For the woman then to be able to consent to the operation and method of anaesthesia, she will need to be given sufficient information about procedures and material risks. Material risks are those that would be seen by the woman to be significant. Risks that the doctors consider would be less significant to the woman need to be addressed only in broad terms (Association of Anaesthetists 1999). On the one hand, the determination of what would be significant or not could be seen to be paternalistic; on the other, it might be considered that the more we expect the woman to understand, the higher the hurdle of perceived autonomy.

Changing Childbirth (Department of Health 1993) was a government report with an ethical basis, particularly with regard to autonomy and justice. Although it stated that women should be able to discuss their wishes and make decisions, it did not bestow rights upon the woman with regard to caesarean section or any other form of care that was in conflict with clinical judgement (Dimond 1999). A 'right', in this sense, suggests that a claim can be made upon others to act in accordance with our wishes (Beauchamp & Childress 1994). Where requested caesarean section is incompatible with the clinical judgement of the obstetrician, there is a moral conflict within the principle of autonomy – that of the woman versus that of the doctor. This might not develop into a moral dilemma if, when considered further in terms of beneficence and non-maleficence, the doctor decided that the woman's reason justified the intervention. The same would apply if the doctor decided that the cost–benefit analysis indicated no intervention unless or until a clinical situation required it. However, if the doctor considered that undertaking the intervention could lead to unnecessary complications, while not undertaking it breached the autonomy of the woman, with which the doctor was not comfortable, then this would be a dilemma.

Cases of enforced caesarean section that occurred in the 1990s resulted in criticism in legal, medical and midwifery circles (Wray 1999). Fovargue & Miola (1998, p. 273) warned that they represented:

...dangerous interventions into the autonomy of pregnancy.

They presumably meant the autonomy of the pregnant woman. Two of these cases resulted in appeal court rulings which upheld the right of the competent woman to self-determination, despite the possible effects on the woman or her fetus (Ashcroft 1998, Re MB 1997, St George's Healthcare NHS Trust v S 1998). Therefore, the law cannot, at least at the present time, legally enforce that a competent pregnant woman should undergo an intervention that she deems inappropriate. Nor can it force doctors to undertake interventions that are against their professional judgement. Therefore, a patient:

...has no absolute right to insist on a specific form of treatment [even when] ... it is clinically indicated (Dimond 1999, p. 515)

It is possible that caesarean section could become an option in areas where the relevant consultants are in favour of it, although resource allocation could be a crucial factor. However, it is unlikely that, in the foreseeable future, it will be offered by all obstetricians. In this case, there is the distinct possibility that some people will consider this to be yet another inequality in services for childbearing women. Perhaps there would be more likelihood of such equal choice if there was the separation of high- and low-risk care, i.e. obstetrics (with obstetric midwifery) and midwifery-led care.

FURTHER DISCUSSION

Autonomy

Downie & Calman (1994, p. 52) define autonomy as follows:

To be an autonomous person is to have the ability to be able to choose for oneself or more extensively to be able to formulate and carry out one's own plans or policies.

Some traits of this principle may be familiar to parents of adolescents, as they are usually involved in encouraging their offspring to '*stand on their own feet*,' '*know what they want*', '*make-up their own minds*' and '*have aims in life*' (Downie & Calman 1994, p. 52).

To be autonomous, then, means being in control of one's life: self-governing and self-ruled. This includes behaving rationally, which in Kant's view is the essence of personhood, and being in control of one's liberty and freedom. Autonomy and freedom are not the same; under the heading of freedom we could say, 'Let them do what they want to', while within autonomy we would say, 'Let them act freely, but they should be able to give reasons for their actions'. The following example puts this into a more practical setting:

> A pregnant woman attends a booking clinic and tells the midwife that she wants a waterbirth. When the midwife asks her why she would like this type of delivery, she states that it is because it is the most natural way to have a baby.

This does not appear to be a rational statement, as it is only 'the most natural way' for amphibians and water mammals. Therefore, further discussion would be necessary for actual autonomous choice to be exercised, as opposed to having the capacity to be autonomous. If the woman stated something similar to:

> *I think that it might provide me with supported mobility, pain relief and a feeling of control*

then it would seem rational and could be planned for.

It is important to consider whether autonomy is a principle that we would wish to uphold. Deontologists may well consider that there can be no negotiation regarding autonomy: it is an intrinsic value of deontology and therefore always a priority. This follows Kant's view that people are ends in themselves and should not be regarded merely as a means to someone else's ends (Benjamin & Curtis 1992). With this in mind, it is important to consider the woman's goals, not the practitioner's. In the given situation, it would be reasonable to assume that the woman's goal was to achieve a successful outcome to her pregnancy, without any pelvic floor damage. The practitioner's goal could have been to keep the woman as a midwife-led case to maintain the figures. In this case, however, it is more likely that he was just as concerned for her general condition as she was for her pelvic floor.

One approach to autonomy is broadly libertarian and assumes that anyone older than a 'toddler' is autonomous, unless mentally defective or possibly emotionally distraught. This is very much a generalisation with no judging of capabilities, although it is considered that autonomy can be lost with age – in cases of senility. This approach suggests that a person's view must be accepted, even in the absence of an acceptable reason or rationality, thus allowing him or her the freedom to make a mistake. This is the perspective often adopted by those on the libertarian end of the political spectrum, and has been supported by philosophers such as Hume, Hobbes and Mill.

Another approach, at the other end of the spectrum, is more rigorous: rationality, reflection and clear judgement are essential factors and autonomy is considered to be a matter of degree rather than an 'all or nothing' capacity. The more rational and deliberate an individual's actions are, the more choice they are allowed; if these elements are weak or absent, then there is the question of whether the decisions should be overridden. Some supporters would consider that someone making decisions based on fear is using an irrational basis; therefore, that person may not be acting autonomously. If that is the case, then some healthcare professionals may believe that decisions should be made for that person, as has previously occurred in cases of unconscious Jehovah's Witnesses requiring a blood transfusion and it being given. It would be fair to say that this approach is no longer widely supported in the case of Jehovah's Witnesses, probably because current professional guidelines are very clear. If advance statements or directives have been made, in identifiable form, then this can be binding on healthcare professionals (Association of Anaesthetists 1999).

In this second approach to autonomy, a person must show that they are doing the right thing for the right reasons, which apparently gives no freedom to make a mistake. Also, consideration should be given as to who decides what is the right reason. Supporters of this approach have included Plato and Rousseau, the latter believing that it is sometimes necessary to force people to be *'free'* – either that or force them to make the choices appropriate to a rational, autonomous individual. Rousseau's approach could result in coercion within the decision-making itself, rather than coercion into the making of a decision.

In this discussion there is concern for the autonomy of the women being cared for during their childbearing experiences, and for that of the health professionals concerned. The majority of the women are healthy. They are undergoing a natural, although not always problem-free, process, one that involves physical, psychological and social change. Therefore the support to which they are entitled involves care within those three aspects, plus educational and, where appropriate, spiritual support. These aspects cannot be totally divorced from one another: there are areas of overlap. For instance, if a woman indicates a psychological problem, such as anxiety regarding pain in labour, which is perfectly understandable, the midwife can discuss the various methods of pain relief available, teach her relaxation exercises and/or arrange for her to attend Preparation for Parenthood classes. In this way she has provided psychological support, education and an insight to the physical support available. In so doing, the midwife will have created an awareness in the woman of possible choices. The degree of awareness created depends, among other things, on the woman's previous knowledge. From discussions with many midwives, as well as through personal experience, the author has determined that women currently appear generally more aware of their bodies and their labour options. This awareness is possibly from the inclusion of health education programmes in schools and from media coverage, such as Caroline provides. Women from all walks of life have expectations of labour, and of themselves and their carers. It is by no means only middle-class women who know what they want, although the level of expectation and understanding may be higher in some cases (Green 1991). Nearly all women at least know what they do not want: they also wish to be involved in decision-making and give rational reasons for their decisions. This surely indicates that these women should be afforded the same respect for autonomy as any other rational person.

Registered or licensed midwives are also autonomous. The midwife can use the knowledge, skills and attitudes acquired during training and subsequent practice (UKCC 1992) in order to achieve the best outcome – that required by the woman as well as the professionals. In practice, however, utilising professional autonomy is very difficult, partly because of the formulation of dogmatic unit policies and procedures. Many of these are very restrictive to the woman's freedom of apparent choice or movement, and to the midwife's practice. Few professionals would argue against the formulation of policies and procedures for the safety of those receiving and giving care. Many do argue, however, that policies should be formulated by a more representative group of professionals. Inflexible, obstetrically oriented and litigation-fearing policies can create a conflict of interests between obstetricians and midwives, which does not provide the best care for the women. Downe (1990) posed the question:

> *Where does the midwife stand legally if a disaster occurs and she has not, on professional grounds, followed the hospital policy?*

From the employment point of view, if the policy was accepted by the health authority, the midwife could have her employment terminated for failure to fulfil her contract. Professionally, however, a midwife cannot plead adherence to hospital policy if accused of misconduct, particularly if this is contrary to up-to-date professional knowledge. The committee responsible for formulating policies should therefore be aware of up-to-date research, be able to evaluate it and be conversant with the needs and requests of the people they are serving. It would appear to be essential for clinical midwives, including a community representative, to be part of this decision-making body. It is not sufficient to have only the senior levels of staff represented; they are often too distant from the specific needs of both the women and the midwives. If it is impossible to include clinical midwives, then a Supervisor of Midwives should serve on the committee, as she is there to preserve the safety and well-being of mothers, babies and midwives. If this well-being is considered at all, then a safe but flexible approach could be taken, in the form of guidelines.

Doctors also have dual autonomy, as people and as practitioners. In their professional lives they are in a position of authority and make decisions regarding management of their patients' conditions and treatments. Ideally, in midwifery and obstetrics, this situation should occur only when a deviation from normal is detected, as midwives are expert practitioners of normal midwifery. In Caroline's situation, she is requesting a deviation from the normal practice and will need to discuss this with the obstetrician, who should then make an autonomous decision in Caroline's best interests. If the obstetrician feels coerced into the caesarean section for some reason, then the degree of autonomy in the decision-making would be questionable.

While autonomy is a principle that we should strive to achieve for ourselves, while respecting and upholding it for others, it must be remembered that generally we live in a society and not in isolation. Just as we are not totally free to do just as we wish, neither are we at liberty to exercise our autonomy at the expense of others.

Paternalism

Paternalism can be on a large scale, as with governmental decisions, or a small scale dealing with individuals. In either case it can be coercive and it is possibly for this reason that antagonism towards it has developed. Examples of large-scale paternalism could be fluoridation of water, where everyone in the area receives the service whether they want it or not, and the law relating to the use of seatbelts. A small-scale example could be the decisions that some healthcare professionals might make on behalf of a patient or client, without seeking or heeding their views.

In teaching ethical principles, paternalism is often portrayed in a negative manner, almost as the opposite of autonomy. This stance can be useful, initially, in trying to instil the importance and application of autonomy, indicating that if one is being paternalistic then the principle of autonomy is not being upheld. However, while that may be true, paternalism is not harmful in intent. On the contrary, it is essentially beneficent and non-maleficent in its application, as those who behave paternalistically do so in the true belief that they know what is best for the client (Beauchamp & Childress 1994).

To be paternalistic is to be very much like a Victorian father, the head of the household who knew what was best for everyone under his roof, particularly his children. There has always been this approach in health care, particularly within the National Health Service. It seems to feel right that it should be part of the package called 'caring': wanting to remove all stresses as being obstacles to getting back to normal. Jones (1996) suggests that healthcare professionals who trained in the days when conformity was the norm are likely to continue this type of practice. Over recent years, however, patients and clients have increasingly been considered partners in their own care; thus paternalism has diminished in some settings, but has not disappeared. The following model and example should help the reader to identify paternalism in health care; and particularly in midwifery.

A healthcare worker (H) is acting paternalistically toward a client (C) only if H's behaviour indicates a belief that:

◆ her action is for C's good;
◆ she is qualified to act on C's behalf;
◆ her action violates, or will violate, a moral rule;
◆ C's good justifies her acting on C's behalf, regardless of any past, present or immediate future informed consent;
◆ C believes, perhaps falsely, that she, herself, knows what is best for her.

(Adapted from Gert & Culver (1979, p. 199)

For example, Karlene has stated that she does not want an episiotomy: she would rather sustain a perineal tear. During the second stage of labour the perineum shows signs of 'buttonholing'. Jane, the midwife, is acting paternalistically towards Karlene only if Jane's behaviour indicates a belief that:

◆ performing an episiotomy is for Karlene's good (i.e. it will prevent a ragged tear);
◆ as a midwife, she is qualified to make these decisions;
◆ performing the episiotomy without consent will violate a moral (as well as legal) rule;
◆ Karlene's good justifies Jane's overruling her wishes;
◆ Karlene believes that she knows what is best for herself.

This is paternalism. If Jane acted the same way but for other reasons, such as:

◆ pressure of time – wanting to get the delivery completed quickly;
◆ not wanting to suture a ragged tear;
◆ lack of belief in women's choice;

this would not be paternalism, it would be a breach of the duty of care. Both situations could result in civil action, but the point is that paternalism may stem from the genuine will to do the best for someone, not necessarily through the will to overpower them. Jones (1996) poses the question of whether autonomy and paternalism are partners or rivals. A personal view is that they are mainly rivals in that those practitioners most likely to be paternalistic are least likely to want to nurture autonomy. However, there are times when clients can make the totally autonomous decision to handover decision-making and responsibility to a professional. In this situation it is right that the professional exercises that softer form of paternalism, as opposed to the aggressive form that exercises power, in which case there would seem to be a partnership of principles.

Consent

...a voluntary, uncoerced decision, made by a sufficiently competent or autonomous person on the basis of adequate information and deliberation, to accept rather than reject some proposed course of action that will affect him or her. (Gillon 1986, p. 113).

This definition, although written some years ago, is very useful as it indicates the relationship between autonomy and consent. If autonomy means being in control of your life, self-governing and self-ruled, then it is essential that the individual is at least a partner in any decision-making process that involves them directly. To be excluded from the process would mean that true consent has not been established.

Health care is one of the most important areas of life in which decisions must be made. People should not feel that they have removed their autonomy with their outdoor clothes, or the closing of an office door. If consent is not sought and gained before carrying out procedures, then the individual has not been allowed to fulfil the above-mentioned essentials of autonomy. In moral terms, therefore, it would seem correct to say that you cannot have one without the other: for consent to be requested, the person must be deemed autonomous; if the person is deemed autonomous then consent is essential, in order to preserve that autonomy.

It is often assumed by the general public that they have to give their consent; this surely is not true consent, rather it is permission under assumed duress. Clients and patients are often made to feel, by well motivated health professionals, that they have no choice. There is always a choice: consent or refusal. Sometimes there is also the possibility of compromise.

It people can give or withhold consent then they have a choice to make. If it is true that they always have a choice, how do they know which decision is the right one? Historically it was assumed that they could not know the answer – hence the paternalistic attitude of the medical, nursing and midwifery professions. More recently, however, there has been a move towards gaining better informed consent, brought about to some extent by certain legal cases, at home and abroad. Achieving informed consent includes giving patients and clients as much information as they need, in understandable terms, in order for them to view their situation accurately and reach their own decision. A number of court cases have held that the giving of adequate information, before requesting consent to procedures, is part of the duty of care; it cannot, therefore, be omitted without a breach of that duty being committed (Dimond 1999).

Gina Boccetti, writing in *Midwifery Matters* (1996, p. 4) stated:

> *The discussions of informed consent that appear in textbooks of medical ethics make it clear that I am not the first to suffer from malignant uncertainty around this issue.*

Discussion with midwives around the country supports Boccetti's view. While English law does not recognise 'informed' consent, as is the case in the USA, neither does it permit ill-informed consent. As stated above, material risks must be discussed and less significant risks must be outlined in broad terms. Failure in the duty to inform could be seen to be a breach in the duty of care, and a civil suit for negligence could ensue.

The definition of consent given above suggests that autonomy and competence are equivalent terms and, until more recent years, this was probably the case. However, Judge Wall (1996) stated:

> *A mentally competent patient has an absolute right to refuse consent to medical treatment for any reason, rational or irrational or for no reason at all, even where that decision will lead to his or her death.*

Competence was then defined by reversal of his definition of incompetence which states that a person lacks competence if incapable of:

◆ comprehending and retaining treatment information;
◆ believing such information;
◆ weighing such information in the balance to make a choice.

Earlier in this book it was stated that civil law is underpinned by ethics, which can be seen by considering different law suits and tracing them back to the principles that were breached. However, where consent is concerned, there now appears to be an ethico-legal confusion. In both ethics and law consent is seen to be fundamental yet, where ethics requires the essential criterion of rationality, law requires only competence, which does not require rationality. With regard to consent, it could now be considered that to insist on ethical practice undermines the law, whereas legal practice could be deemed to be unethical.

Consent, as discussed so far, relates to the adult. It also relates to most 16–18 year olds, where the *Family Law Reform Act 1969* allows for minors of such age, if deemed competent by adult standards, to consent or refuse for themselves. This should not mean, however, that minors who are under 16 years of age are at the mercy of the professionals with whom they come in contact. It is usual for parents or other legal guardians to protect their children. They can refuse what they deem to be unnecessary or harmful and they can offer proxy consent, in the best interests of the child, where investigation or treatment is required.

Since 1985, however, there has been the opportunity for young people under the age of 16 years to consent to treatment, and in theory refuse it, for themselves (Bloy 1996). This was brought about by the well known Gillick case (1985). Although the case itself related to provision of contraception, the principles of 'Gillick competence' can be applied to any healthcare issue involving male or female minors. To be deemed 'Gillick competent' in a childbearing situation, a girl must be able to understand the situation that she is in; she must understand the options open to her, once they have been explained to her; and she must understand the possible consequences of each of these options. This is quite an expectation and, some would say, greater than what we actually expect of an adult. Perhaps it is intended to create an added safeguard. It must also be recognised, however, that, although a minor may offer consent or refusal, the decision can be overridden if it is thought to be in the child's best interests (Bloy 1996). The cynical view is that the child can consent to anything but, should she refuse a course of action considered appropriate by a health professional, she will undoubtedly be deemed incompetent.

It would be interesting to contemplate what would happen if a 15-year-old girl chose not to have screening for fetal abnormality.

Ethically the girl should not be treated as a means to another's end. The 'other' could be the fetus, or the professionals or parents who want to know what lies ahead. To enforce the screening tests would be putting a non-person, or the wishes of others, before the wishes of the girl; this would surely be unethical practice.

Regardless of the age of the client, where there is failure to obtain consent before 'touching', the person is entitled to sue in the civil court for 'trespass against the person'; this equates to the crime of *battery*.

APPLYING THE THEORIES TO CAROLINE'S CASE

Utilitarian views

Act-utilitarians would examine the benefits that might be promoted by Caroline being granted her request, not only to Caroline, but to the professionals, the service and society. They would also consider the possible risks involved and would aim to achieve a greater balance of benefit over risk. Autonomy is an extrinsic value to utilitarians, and is therefore non-essential if the consequences were such that, by respecting the principle, less good would be achieved than by not respecting it.

For Caroline, the consequences of allowing her request could include a fulfilled woman with a healthy baby and no perineal trauma. However, the caesarean section could result in short- and long-term morbidity, even mortality in some cases, for the mother and baby, and she may not maintain a perfect pelvic floor. For the professionals, the benefits and risks will depend on the quality of outcome; a poor outcome could result in some form of litigation. For the service, the cost of the caesarean section and the aftercare, even if all is well, will decrease the financial resources available for caring for other mothers and babies. Where such expenditure is required through necessity, this would be acceptable; however, if it is by choice and not necessity then it would be less acceptable. For society, it could create the impression that any demand will be met, or it could undermine women's ability to carry out a natural function, thus creating fear. It is quite possible, based on the limited analysis here, that act-utilitarians would favour refusal of Caroline's request.

Rule-utilitarians would also wish to achieve the greatest benefit for the greatest number of people. They might look at the overall picture in general terms, considering the risk–benefit analysis of women in general requesting caesarean section. It is quite likely that they would make the same final decision as the act-utilitarians.

Deontological views

The Kantian view would initially consider that failure to uphold Caroline's autonomous decision would result in a failure of duty. Consideration of the universalisation principle, however, could well indicate a failed duty if her request was fulfilled, as performing caesarean sections on all pregnant women, without justification, would not be a rational action.

Mill's view of Caroline's individuality, or autonomy, would be that maintaining her individual stance would be acceptable as long as it did not compromise the individual stance of others (Beauchamp & Childress 1994). For instance, assume that Caroline's obstetrician is not in favour of caesarean section on demand, but remember that Caroline is the central figure in this professional relationship. Where Kant's initial opinion could well be that she should be allowed her choice, Mill would probably state that she cannot insist on her choice if it will compromise the obstetrician.

A pluralist would probably find conflict between beneficence and non-maleficence but could be swayed by their own view of the relative safety of caesarean section. However, if the duty of justice was seen to be first in the priority ordering of the duties, then the justice of this woman having as much right to her choice as anyone else might be the deciding factor. It should be remembered that pluralists would be looking at their duties to Caroline, not to anyone else.

REFERENCES

Al-Mufti R, McCarthy A, Fisk N M 1997 Survey of obstetricians' personal preference and discretionary practice. European Journal of Obstetrics, Gynecology, and Reproductive Biology 73:1–4

Amu O, Rajendren S, Bolaji I I 1998 Maternal choice alone should not determine method of delivery. (Should doctors perform an elective caesarean section on request?) British Medical Journal 317 (156):463–465

Ashcroft B 1998 Court-ordered caesarean sections: a midwife's dilemma. British Journal of Midwifery 6(4):259–261

Association of Anaesthetists of Great Britain and Ireland 1999 Information and consent for anaesthesia. AAGBI, London

Beauchamp T L, Childress J F 1994 Principles of biomedical ethics, 4th edn. Oxford University Press, Oxford

Benjamin M, Curtis J 1992 Ethics in nursing, 3rd edn. Oxford University Press, Oxford

Bloy D J 1996 Child law. Cavendish, London

Boccetti G 1996 Informed consent? Midwifery Matters 70:3–5

Department of Health 1993 Changing childbirth. Report of the Expert Maternity Group. HMSO, London

Dimond B 1999 Is there a legal right to choose a caesarean? British Journal of Midwifery 7(8):515–518

Downe S 1990 Conflict of interests. Nursing Times 86(47):14

Downie R S, Calman K C 1994 Healthy respect. Oxford Medical Publications, Oxford

Dyer C 1997 Court of Appeal decision. British Medical Journal 314:993

Gert B, Culver C M 1979 The justification of paternalism. In: Medicine and moral philosophy–readings from philosophy and public affairs. Princeton University Press, Princeton, p 199

Gillick v West Norfolk Area Health Authority. 1985 3 All E R 402

Gillon R 1986 Philosophical medical ethics. John Wiley, Chichester

Green J M 1991 Expectations, experiences and psychological outcomes of childbirth. Birth 17(1):15–24

Fovargue S, Miola J 1998 Policing pregnancy: implications of the Attorney-General's reference (no. 3 of 1994). Cited in Grubb A, Medical Law Review 6(3):265–296

Jones H 1996 Autonomy and paternalism: partners or rivals? British Journal of Nursing 5(6):378–381

Montgomery J 1997 Health care law. Oxford University Press, Oxford

Page L 1999 Caesarean birth: the kindest cut? British Journal of Midwifery 7(5):296

Paterson-Brown S 1998 Yes, as long as the woman is fully informed. (Should doctors perform an elective caesarean section on request?) British Medical Journal 317(7156):462–463

Re M B 1997 8 Med L R 217

Robinson J 1998 Caesarean section: women's choice. British Journal of Midwifery 6(10):669

Robinson J 1999 The demand for caesareans: fact or fiction. British Journal of Midwifery 7(5):306

St George's Healthcare NHS Trust v S 1998 3 All E R 673

UKCC 1992 Scope of professional practice. UKCC, London

UKCC 1996 Guidelines for professional practice. UKCC, London

Wall, Judge 1996 Tameside and Glossop Acute Services Trust v CH 1 F C R 753

Wray E 1999 Court authorised caesarean sections. British Journal of Midwifery 7(7):443–446

SUGGESTED ADDITIONAL READING

Ashcroft B 1998 Choices in childbirth: myth or reality. British Journal of Midwifery 6(8):502–506

Beauchamp T L, Childress J F 1994 Respect for autonomy. In: Beauchamp TL, Childress JF. Principles of biomedical ethics, 4th edn. Oxford University Press, Oxford, ch 3

Draper H 1996 Women, forced caesareans and antenatal responsibilities. Journal of Medical Ethics 22:327–333

Goldbeck-Wood S 1997 Women's autonomy in childbirth. British Medical Journal 314:1143–1144

Lewinson H 1996 Choices in childbirth: areas of conflict. In: Frith L (ed) Ethics and midwifery. Issues in contemporary practice. Butterworth–Heinemann, Oxford, p 36

Malyon D 1998 Transfusion-free treatment of Jehovah's Witnesses: respecting the autonomous patient's rights. Journal of Medical Ethics 24:302–307

Muramoto O 1998a Bioethics of the refusal of blood by Jehovah's Witnesses: part 1. Should bioethical deliberation consider dissidents' views? Journal of Medical Ethics 24:233–230

Muramoto O 1998b Bioethics of the refusal of blood by Jehovah's Witnesses: part 2. A novel approach based on rational non-interventional paternalism. Journal of Medical Ethics 24:295–301

Savulescu J, Myomer R W 1997 Should informed consent be based on rational beliefs? Journal of Medical Ethics 23:282–288

Symon A 1997 Consent and choice: the rights of the patients. British Journal of Midwifery 5(5):256–258

8

Conscientious objection to participation in abortion

Angela was 28 years old, married to Jo and in her second pregnancy, having had a son three years ago. All was well with her pregnancy until an ultrasound scan (USS) was performed at 25 weeks of gestation. This scan had been planned for 20 weeks of gestation but had been delayed, first because of a holiday that had already been booked, then because her son was ill, and then because of a technical problem in the USS department.

Angela was not concerned by the delay as she felt certain that all was well. When she eventually had the scan, it was discovered that the fetus had sustained an intraventricular haemorrhage (IVH). Discussions with relevant doctors suggested that the prognosis was good but it was agreed that serial scans should be performed, in order to observe any significant changes. Unfortunately, at 33 weeks' gestation, another IVH had occurred and the prognosis was now poor. Angela and Jo were advised of the situation and were offered termination of pregnancy as an option open to them. They discussed the procedures that would be necessary with the obstetrician and then went home to discuss the devastating news.

Angela and Jo decided to have the pregnancy terminated. At 34 weeks of gestation, Angela presented herself at the USS department with Jo there to support her. Angela was given mifepristone orally and then, with the aid of the USS equipment, feticide by intracardiac injection of potassium chloride was carried out. Angela was not prepared for the fact that she would be aware of the moment of death of her baby. He had moved violently, then suddenly stopped. Angela and Jo were taken to the delivery suite for continuation with the termination of the pregnancy; however, because she was very distressed, it was some hours before the process was continued.

As there had been a time delay already, it was agreed to wait until the start of the next shift, so that there was as much continuity for Angela as possible. However, when the midwives arrived, no-one was willing to take on the case. Some members of staff had always avoided termination of pregnancy cases because of moral concerns, while others felt that they could not be involved in termination at such a late gestation.

None of them had ever committed their views to paper for inclusion in their files. The midwifery unit manager stated that the midwives must care for Angela as if she had experienced a spontaneous intrauterine fetal death (IUD). Some midwives felt that this was a very insensitive response and asked for advice from a Supervisor of Midwives in another part of the unit.

The Supervisor advised that the midwives would have to care for Angela, with appropriate sensitivity, on this occasion. She also stated that, after the delivery was over, she would discuss the matter further with any midwife who might find it beneficial. Two midwives offered to care for Angela. After delivery of the baby, a boy weighing 2.4 kg, the parents and the midwives were very distressed, not least because there were a number of marks on the baby's chest which indicated that a number of attempts to carry out the intracardiac injection had been made.

A few days after Angela left the unit, she wrote to the midwifery manager commending the two midwives for the care and attention given to her, Jo and their son.

QUESTIONS FOR CONSIDERATION BY THE READER

1. Is it right to carry out abortion at this late gestation?
2. Could Angela have been better prepared for what to expect during the procedure?
3. Were the midwives at liberty to refuse to care for Angela?
4. What could the midwifery manager and Supervisor of Midwives do to prevent a recurrence of this situation?

QUESTION 1: IS IT RIGHT TO CARRY OUT ABORTION AT THIS LATE GESTATION?

The *Abortion Act 1967* was initially passed to stop, or at least radically reduce, the sometimes devastating effects of illegal abortion. Such abortions were sometimes self-induced, but often the result of intervention by 'back street' abortionists. Some abortionists were doctors or nurses, some had no proper knowledge but genuinely tried to help the women who came to them, while others were opportunists who made money at the expense of vulnerable women of all ages. The victims suffered varying degrees of morbidity and even death, having paid large sums of money for the privilege.

This Act stated the broad circumstances under which termination of a pregnancy could take place. Because of the link with the *Infant Life (Preservation) Act 1929*, which protected the life of the viable fetus, abortion could not take place after the 28th gestational week. In practice, many obstetricians had personal cut-off points prior to 28 weeks, in some cases because the dates were questionable.

The Abortion Act was amended by the *Human Fertilisation and Embryology Act 1990*. Among other changes, it now states an upper gestational limit of 24 weeks for the circumstances that were covered by the earlier Act. However, termination of pregnancy was made legal at any gestation, up to birth (Morgan & Lee 1991), in certain extreme circumstances:

◆ to prevent grave permanent injury to the physical or mental health of the woman;
◆ where there is risk to the life of the woman;
◆ where there is substantial risk that the child would suffer from physical or mental abnormalities that would cause serious handicap.

In the first two categories above, the intention would obviously be to do the best for the fetus, aiming to have a good outcome for both mother and baby. However, as Angela's fetus was considered to have a poor prognosis following the second IVH, it would be considered that there would be serious mental and physical handicap to a child born alive. Therefore, this case came within the grounds for legal termination of pregnancy at any gestation, with a view to the baby not surviving.

Legally, abortion is allowed at this gestation and, as the fetus is not legally a person until separated from its mother, it has no legal rights normally attributed to persons. This in itself creates an ethical issue for, if the fetus had not been at risk of serious disability, it would not have been legal to terminate its life. This could be seen by some people as discrimination against potential persons with disabilities. It is also said by some people that action of this nature devalues the lives of those who already live with disabilities of varying degrees, and appears to have eugenic undertones.

It could be seen by others that, if the child were born alive, his life would be such that he would have:

> ...little or no prospect of meaningful interaction with others or the environment ... no reasonable person would want to lead such a life, nor impose on a doctor a duty to strive to bring it about. (Royal College of Paediatrics and Child Health 1997, p. 17)

In which case, if the child were born alive, he would probably be allowed to die if the parents and staff considered this to be appropriate. Therefore, little would be achieved by delivering him alive, except more suffering perhaps. Viewed in this way, it can be seen that the *Abortion Act 1967* (as amended) has made provision in pregnancy for what would be termed euthanasia in independent life. This is one of the reasons why some people cannot condone such practice.

The *Abortion Act 1967*, in its original and amended forms, allows a woman to do what she believes is ethically right for her and her family at that time, in those circumstances. As the fetus is not a person, our ethical considerations should be concerned first with the woman and her family, not the fetus (see Further discussion). Angela had been given information about the condition of her baby. She was given the options of continuing with the pregnancy, with the future predicted to be very poor, or of terminating it. She and Jo took time to discuss the situation and make a decision. This would suggest that Angela was acting as autonomously as she could in the circumstances (see Ch. 7 Autonomy and consent).

With regard to beneficence and non-maleficence, Angela might be considered to have greater benefit and less long-term harm by undergoing the termination, rather than having the trauma of caring for a very disabled baby for his life-time. On the other hand, it could be that Angela will suffer long-term guilt and experience none of the joy of caring for her son, whatever his condition. It is possible that Angela and Jo made their decision based on the benefit, harm and justice for their first son. It is well known that babies and children with major disabilities take a lot of time and effort. This could leave the parents with little time and energy for the existing child.

QUESTION 2: COULD ANGELA HAVE BEEN BETTER PREPARED FOR WHAT TO EXPECT DURING THE PROCEDURE?

While it is difficult to know how much detail Angela and Jo were given, it would be reasonably safe to consider that the *procedures* would have included the feticide and induction of labour, at least in broad terms. What they might not have been given were the exact effects of the procedures, other than to say that the first procedure was to ensure that their baby was dead before the labour was started.

It is quite possible that the person outlining the procedures did not know what Angela would experience. Perhaps different fetuses react in different ways. Perhaps the fact that a number of attempts had been made to get the needle into the fetal chest had some bearing on its response. Perhaps that unit had not undertaken this procedure on a fetus of that gestation before, therefore they could not know what information to give Angela. Only if they did know could we say that Angela should have been better informed.

If there was the possibility of women being given a light general anaesthetic while the intracardiac injection was given, to prevent their awareness of the moment of death, would they take that opportunity? It is possible that some women would refuse it, feeling that they should suffer the ordeal as a punishment for the decision they have made.

QUESTION 3: WERE THE MIDWIVES AT LIBERTY TO REFUSE TO CARE FOR ANGELA?

In general terms, midwives are not at liberty to refuse to care for any woman (UKCC 1996, 1998). However, just as the law allows for women to do what is ethically right for them with regard to abortion, it has also provided healthcare professionals with the legal right to do what they consider to be ethically right for themselves (Jones 1999). Both the initial and the amended versions of the Act allow for conscientious objection to participation in abortion, covered by Section 4. This section states:

> *(1) Subject to subsection (2) of this section, no person shall be under any duty, whether by contract or by any statutory or other*

legal requirement, to participate in any treatment authorised by this Act to which he has a conscientious objection:

Provided that in any legal proceedings the burden of proof of conscientious objection shall rest upon the person claiming to rely on it.

This subsection states 'he' but it also relates to female healthcare workers. It also expects that the member of staff should be prepared to disclose their objection, and makes it quite clear that the midwife cannot be bound by the legal duty of care, in normal circumstances. The *Code of Professional Conduct* (UKCC 1992, clause 8), in line with the Act, also allows for practitioners to express their conscientious objection. Section 4 of the Act continues:

(2) Nothing in subsection (1) of this section shall affect any duty to participate in treatment which is necessary to save the life or to prevent grave permanent injury to the physical or mental health of a pregnant woman.

In other words, even though a midwife might be excused from caring for Angela on conscientious grounds, she must be prepared to care for her – as with any other woman – in the event of emergencies such as haemorrhage, cardiac arrest or eclamptic fit. Here the midwife would have a duty of care if emergency assistance was requested.

To be able to claim exemption from caring for any woman undergoing termination of pregnancy on the grounds of conscientious objection, it is expected that the midwife will have notified her manager, in writing, before any particular case emerges. Dimond (1999) suggests that the objection should be raised at interview. However, unless termination of pregnancy features in the job description, midwives do not have to discuss the issue at interview, any more than their plans for a family or organisation of childcare. If the matter was raised by a panel member, when not in the job description, and the midwife was not appointed, the midwife could view the interview as being discriminatory. It should also be remembered that people can change their views regarding many aspects of care, including abortion, long after taking up post. For instance, in a television documentary regarding extrauterine fetal surgery, the American obstetrician Joseph Bruner stated that his work with repair of spina bifida has changed his view of abortion: he is no longer convinced that it is acceptable (Bruner 1999).

In the situation under discussion, as none of the midwives had notified a conscientious objection before this case, none of them had the legal or professional right to refuse to care for her. Common sense and sensitivity, however, suggest that it would be to no-one's advantage to force someone into caring for Angela against their will, so long as there is a volunteer. In this case there were two, which served as a means of support for the midwives as well as Angela and Jo. It also shows lack of understanding and sensitivity for the manager to state that Angela should be cared for as if she had experienced a spontaneous IUD. Angela requires her carers to understand some of what she has gone through and has yet to experience. Also, the midwives with conscientious objections would be adding to their moral compromise to pretend that this was not abortion.

Healthcare professionals are expected to be non-judgemental in their care. By notifying a conscientious objection before a specific case arises, there can be no claim of judgemental practice, as there is no specific client to be judged.

QUESTION 4: WHAT COULD THE MIDWIFERY MANAGER AND SUPERVISOR OF MIDWIVES DO TO PREVENT A RECURRENCE OF THIS SITUATION?

It would seem appropriate, under the circumstances, that both the manager and Supervisor could start by debriefing the midwives who were on duty during the time that Angela was on the delivery suite, starting with the two who cared for her.

The unit in question obviously needs to educate their midwives with regard to notification of conscientious objection to participation in abortion. The manager is the person responsible for ensuring that the appropriate number of staff are on duty, with the relevant skill mix, in order to carry out the Trust's business. It could be said, therefore, that she is a little too close to the staffing situation to be involved in counselling midwives with regard to this issue. It might be more appropriate for the Supervisor to do this, or the relevant Supervisors for the individual midwives. Care is needed in cases where the Supervisors are also managers, to ensure that the moral well-being of the midwives is being served at the same time as ensuring care for patients.

It is also evident that the unit needs guidelines in respect of such cases, preferably before another situation presents itself. It would be useful to have a multidisciplinary team approach to writing the guidelines. There could be representation from midwives, managers, Supervisors, obstetricians, ultrasonographers and paediatricians, to ensure that all professional parties are represented. It would seem appropriate, on the one hand, to invite someone like Angela to participate but, on the other hand, this would probably be too painful. In this case someone from the support group Support Around Termination For Abnormality (SATFA) could be asked to represent the clients.

FURTHER DISCUSSION

The case in this chapter relates to late gestation abortion for fetal abnormality. However, some Trusts have developed their women's services in such a way that all abortions, for whatever reasons, are undertaken within the obstetric service. This means that midwives and students are required to undertake this care. This section will not address the issues surrounding all abortion, but will concentrate on second and third trimester abortion for fetal abnormality. Some of the points, however, would transfer to any case of abortion, particularly those relating to conscientious objection.

The following discussion will include some aspects of screening, as this is the starting point for late abortion, conscientious objection, maternal versus fetal rights with regard to abortion, and consideration of feticide before induction of labour.

Screening for fetal abnormality

Modern technology has provided society with the opportunity of diagnosing a pregnancy before the woman has missed her first menstrual period – a very different picture to the days when women waited until at least two periods had been missed before seeking confirmation of pregnancy. This earlier confirmation, coupled with advanced technology, provides greater opportunity for investigating the state of the fetus, should this be required.

It would seem reasonable to determine what is meant by *fetal screening*. It sounds as though all fetuses are checked, from head to toe, inside and out, to detect any possible abnormality. This is obviously not the case; at least, it is obvious to those who have regular dealings with such matters, but not necessarily to the general public. It is possible that the public expects more of technology and the National Health Service than is actually available. The author will accept the old but useful definition of screening provided by Cuckle & Wald (1984, p. 1) as:

> *...the identification, among apparently healthy individuals, of those who are sufficiently at risk of a specific disorder to justify a subsequent diagnostic test or procedure, or in certain circumstances, direct preventive action.*

Screening is generally the preliminary step towards the detection of disorders that may require further investigation. It can be used where specific disorders are anticipated in high-risk individuals, for instance genetic disorders, or it can be used with a large sample of the population, as is carried out for rubella immunity in pregnancy. In itself, screening is not diagnosis. Diagnosis is the identification of a disease or anomaly which may be assisted by the results of screening. These terms are, therefore, not interchangeable.

There are basically two types of fetal screening. The first type deals with the routine screening offered to all mothers who attend clinics early enough for it to be carried out. The second type relates to the woman whose fetus is deemed to be at greater risk of genetic disorders or congenital abnormality. This would include:

◆ those who have previously had babies with certain abnormalities;
◆ where there is a family history of such problems;
◆ where either the woman or her partner has an inheritable disease – or one that could create other abnormalities in the baby, as with diabetes mellitus;
◆ where the woman has contracted diseases such as rubella or toxoplasmosis during early pregnancy; or
◆ where the woman is aged 35 years or older, when it is considered more likely that chromosomal abnormality could occur.

Antenatal screening tests are specific; however, they do not always directly screen the fetus. Some of them test the woman for conditions that could adversely affect her or her fetus in pregnancy, labour or infancy/childhood. Testing for human immunodeficiency virus status would be included in this category. Women can be offered the opportunity of being tested with no obligation to accept. There is obviously much to debate on this issue, but it will not be continued here.

Other tests are specific to the fetal condition and these include: maternal serum screening, ultrasonographic scanning, chorionic villus sampling, amniocentesis, Doppler assessments, biophysical profiling and fetoscopy.

When adverse results are received, although decisions rest with the couple alone, it would be a mistake to assume that outside influences are ignored. Apart from listening to professional points of view, couples often consider the opinions of family and friends. If they feel that their child would be poorly received, this might aid their decision to abort the fetus. On the other hand, if they feel that there would be positive and supportive reaction, then they may be able to cope with the possible trials ahead. Their general socialisation, from childhood onwards, would also influence their decision-making (e.g. education, religious beliefs and media portrayal of disabilities in general). Down's syndrome has fared particularly well since the MENCAP campaign of the late 1970s and early 1980s, with society being better educated to accept people with this disorder. Anecdotal evidence from midwives across the UK suggests that there has been an increase in women deciding against screening tests. Also, where screening is undertaken and Down's syndrome is a high risk, or further diagnostic procedures confirm it, more women are choosing to continue with the pregnancy and appropriate preparation.

Some women choose to be tested with no intention of having an abortion, regardless of the results. They may be choosing to know of any detectable disability in order to grieve for the loss of what might have been, giving better opportunity for developing interaction after delivery. Also it gives time to prepare for what is facing them and how they are going to cope with it.

It should be remembered that we do not make decisions in a vacuum; we are often influenced and constrained by the views of others. Family and friends were mentioned previously in this respect, but society in general imposes opinions, particularly with regard to the perceived value of life of disabled people. These opinions are often voiced through the media, but they are also expressed verbally and non-verbally in streets, shops and other public places. In some cases comments are made during conversations, in others it may be the sight of a disabled child or adult that causes comment or facial expression. The attitudes exhibited range from pity, through a variety of others, to repulsion. The knowledge that this will undoubtedly occur at some time will be in the minds of many people facing this type of decision, with consideration of whether they can cope with either extreme.

Society's views of screening tests for fetal abnormality could be creating a roller-coaster effect. The test is performed, an abnormality is discovered, therefore termination of pregnancy is accepted or even expected; this is based on the perceived quality of life as opposed to the value of life (see Ch. 10). This is a disposable age: if something is imperfect, it is thrown away and replaced. It is possible that this could eventually happen with minor fetal defects. Society may even develop expectations that all women at risk should be tested, with no freedom of choice.

Another possible problem with screening and diagnostic tests is that, while the test may be performed in order to diagnose or rule out certain disorders, it is possible that it could detect something that was not previously considered. This could create a dilemma for the doctors, particularly if the prognosis is unknown or there is a good chance that the anomaly will not produce a major problem, such as an extra Y chromosome. The author is not suggesting that Richards' (1988, p. 176) hypothetical thoughts should be adopted:

Perhaps we need to discipline ourselves to ignore information that arrives by serendipity.

Rather, it is being highlighted that, unless good counselling has taken place regarding this possibility, the woman/couple may not be prepared for the actual findings.

Conscientious objection

Abortion is a very sensitive subject which can stimulate passionate responses across the spectrum of society. The intention here is to indicate some of the major points of the argument related to conscientious objection, not to enter the early abortion debate.

For some people the objection would be of a religious nature, particularly relating to the sanctity of life. Others might feel that they would be morally compromised, regardless of whether they have any religious views. Burnard & Chapman (1993) state that it is important to know the difference between objections based on strongly held principles and those specific situations where there is more of a professional disagreement.

In Angela's case, it would appear that some midwives were disagreeing with the professional judgement of conducting a termination of pregnancy at such a late gestation, rather than having a general objection to abortion. Others, particularly those mentioned as avoiding terminations based on moral concerns, probably fit into the group most likely to notify conscientious objections once they know what to do.

Whether the conscientious objections stem from religious or moral views, the underlying principles usually relate to the issue of killing the fetus. Some people would go so far as to state that it is murder; others use euphemisms such as 'taking a life' or 'destroying a potential life'. Those with objections on religious grounds feel that they would be compromised in the eyes of their God, while those with no religious beliefs are more likely to feel a personal sense of moral compromise.

One reason for objection is the view that an embryo/fetus is a human life from conception, and that all human life must be preserved; this is the sanctity of life principle (see Ch. 10). This view does not necessarily assume that the fetus is a person, just that it is human and alive. Some people accept that it is human in genetic make-up and alive in the sense that it is not dead, but they would not attach any moral value to it until it is truly alive by surviving on its own. Mahowald (1995, p. 201) indicates this view:

...it is consistently recognized that fetuses exist only in relationship to women who are inevitably affected by decisions regarding them.

However, there are others who would respond that fetuses are inevitably affected by decisions made by and on behalf of the women carrying them.

The central point of argument within the abortion debate seems to be the joint issues of personhood and the right to life. Those who are against abortion – often known as the pro-life lobby – view the fetus as a person with an absolute right to life, hence their view that abortion is killing and therefore morally wrong (Palmer 1999). Those who are not against abortion – the pro-choice lobby – argue that the fetus is not a person and therefore has no independent right to life (Mahowald 1995, Palmer 1999). Considerations surrounding the central argument of personhood and the right to life, include when life begins and the notion of 'potential' (Morgan & Lee 1991). There is then the consideration of the rights of the fetus: whether it has any and how they fit in with the rights of the woman.

Life could be said to begin at the moment of birth, or at least when the first breath of air is inhaled; many people are comfortable with this notion. Others, however, would say that that is the beginning of independent life, but that actual life begins before this. For midwives who are familiar with those hours of labour before the beginning of independent life, it would probably be very difficult to consider that birth is the actual starting point of life. They have, by various means, been monitoring the life of that fetus in the form of its heart rate and movements throughout the labour. In fact, other midwives have been monitoring the fetus by similar activities since half-way through the pregnancy, if not before. We cannot say that there was no life there then. So when did it start? It is obvious that by following this train of thought back in time we would inevitably come back to the moment of conception, or for some people the journey would extend beyond that to the living cells that started the process: the gametes. This gives us two extremes: at the earliest point we have biological life, and at the final point, birth, we have independent life. Many people would say that taking either of the extremes would be unjust for the woman and for the fetus. Palmer (1999) suggests that there has occurred a blurring of the distinction between the fetus and the neonate, mainly due to the advances in fetal photography. Indeed there is now a subspecialty of fetal medicine within obstetrics, creating patient status for the fetus, thus giving credibility to the notion of fetal rights. As fetal development is continuous, viability seems to be the point of compromise, which can be accepted from a legal stance but is still not acknowledged by all from a moral perspective.

In the UK viability is deemed to be 24 weeks of gestation, hence this is the cut-off point for most abortions. While the removal of a time limit for abortion for fetal abnormality has relieved the pressures regarding the timing of tests and receipt of results, it has created other problems. Some healthcare professionals who accept abortion before viability, have greater difficulty accepting the idea, morally, once the fetus is viable. The longer the gestation, the greater the degree of anxiety experienced by greater numbers of people, as late termination seems more like infanticide than abortion (Warnock 1998). This has nothing to do with making judgements on the women concerned; practitioners are well aware that these women have made heart-searching decisions to abort wanted babies (Andrews 1997). Rather it is to do with the perceived moral compromise of the practitioners themselves, the effects of which can be devastating.

To determine whether or not a fetus should be considered a person, Purdy & Tooley (1999, p. 46) maintain the broad thrust of Tooley's deliberations from the late 1970s. Their view is:

> ...an organism can have a right to life only if it now possesses, or possessed at some time in the past, the capacity to have a desire for continued existence.

It is possible that a fetus could be such an organism, particularly as gestation progresses, as the fact that it has a brain suggests that it has the capacity for brain function. When we consider the poor uterine environments in which some fetuses survive, it could be said that they seem to have survival instincts, which could be seen as a desire for continued existence. If the fetus is deemed not to fit this criterion, then it could be said that a newborn baby is no different and therefore does not have the right to life. Purdy & Tooley (1999, p. 46) go on to say:

> An organism cannot satisfy this requirement unless it is a person, that is, a continuing subject of experience and other mental states, and unless it has the capacity for self-consciousness – where an organism is self-conscious only if it recognizes that it is itself a person.

A fetus could be seen to be a continuing subject of experience and other mental states (we know that fetuses respond to music, their mothers' voices and adrenaline levels); what it presumably cannot do is recognise itself as a person. For those readers with experience of children, contemplate at what age children become aware of themselves as persons. This part of their statement could suggest that a baby is not a person until it is well developed and therefore has no right to life. Others would argue that the fetus has the potential for all that would class it as a person, and therefore it should be treated with the same respect as a person and should be granted the right to life.

Having determined the background to why people may notify a conscientious objection to participation in abortion, we need to explore exactly what it is from which they are exempt. Verbal reports indicate that some managers insist that midwives are exempt only from the process of feticide, where it is used, or insertion of the pessaries used to start the labour. There appears to be confusion as to what constitutes termination of pregnancy. However, if we consider, as a civil court might do, what any reasonable person would consider to be the termination, it would probably be from the start of the process to the clearing away of the products of conception (Jones 1999, Dimond 1999). If so, this is what the midwife should be exempt from, except, as stated earlier, in the case of a life-threatening emergency.

Some healthcare professionals object to taking part in any stage of the care of women undergoing abortion, at any gestation. They feel that they should not deal with referral letters or admission procedures. While it is possible to see their point of view, it should also be seen that these procedures are no different from what is required for any patient or client; therefore, refusal amounts to being judgemental. The content of the letter or the reason for the admission should not influence the staff. A midwife must be prepared to care for the woman up to the start of the process and to care for her postnatally, at all times with respect.

The Royal College of Midwives (1997) has produced a statement on conscientious objection, which should have helped midwives to understand their position with regard to termination of pregnancy. Instead, it created greater confusion as it stated on the front page:

> ...the conscientious objection clause should only include direct involvement in the procedure of terminating pregnancy. Thus all midwives should be prepared to care for women before, during and after termination...

Perhaps this is where the previously mentioned managers got their ideas.

Maternal versus fetal rights

During the 1990s there was rising concern regarding the dilemma relating to maternal versus fetal rights. Legally the dilemma should not exist as the fetus has very limited rights. The rights afforded refer to the subjects of: inheritance, congenital disability and personal injury. There is also some protection afforded by the *Infant Life (Preservation) Act 1929* and the *Abortion Act 1967* (as amended). However, the protection afforded the fetus after 24 weeks could be said to be limited. The protection includes that only those with serious anomalies can be aborted with no intention of them surviving. This gives rise to moral concerns regarding the inequality of status between fetuses with anomalies and those without. Also, Noonan (1999, p. 43) states:

> *Experience, which teaches us that even the most seriously incapacitated prefer living to dying, is ignored.*

For some practitioners, the apparently eugenic position of abortion for fetal abnormality adds to their moral disquiet.

The apparent conflict between maternal and fetal rights is of a moral nature. If we agree to consider the fetus to have moral rights, then we must consider what those rights are and whose rights would be considered to be paramount in cases of conflict. Perhaps one right would be the right not to be harmed. Women could find themselves legally restricted to certain 'dos' and 'don'ts' during pregnancy and labour. Areas that might be considered in pregnancy are diet, smoking, alcohol intake, travel, type of employment, attendance at Preparation for Parenthood classes; in labour it could be place, method of pain relief, and so on. This would be a removal of the woman's rights and would be placing the worth of a fetus above that of an already independent living person.

It could be envisaged that many people, professional and non-professional, would applaud the suggestion of fetal rights with regard to harmful practices. This could, however, be the start of the slippery slope, where consideration of fetal rights rapidly results in the over-ruling of maternal rights. Most women, however committed to their unborn babies, would not wish to see a police state for pregnancy.

Let us assume that rights have been given to the fetus. In the case in question we would have Angela's right to terminate her pregnancy, on the grounds that her baby would be badly damaged from the IVHs he suffered in utero, versus the fetus's right to life. The right to a life of what quality? Quality of life is difficult to determine for another adult (see Ch. 10), so it would be even more difficult to predict for a child, particularly when the exact nature of the disabilities would not be known immediately. If the baby was born alive with major disabilities, then Angela and the team of carers would have to make decisions about treatment (see Ch. 10). The decisions could result in the baby's eventual death. In this case, it would appear that Angela has probably decided, in her baby's best interests, to make those decisions before the baby has to suffer both the disability and the treatment.

However just and honourable Angela's decision was, this would not help to prevent the moral compromise of the midwives with a conscientious objection to participation in the process.

Live birth following termination of pregnancy

When we consider the early gestations at which preterm labour can result in babies being born alive, albeit not without damage in some cases, we must consider the possible outcomes of abortion where feticide is not carried out beforehand. In spontaneous preterm labour, or induction of labour preterm because of a condition in the mother (still termination of pregnancy), the labour is monitored so that intervention can take place if the fetus becomes distressed or the mother's condition deteriorates. With abortion for fetal abnormality, the intention is that the fetus should not survive, so the labour will not be monitored from the fetus's point of view. This suggests that we are intending to let the fetus suffer the labour to the point of its death. This does not seem very humane. It seems unjust to think that we could have one preterm fetus being observed and cared for in one room, while another of a similar or later gestation in the next room is being treated by something akin to torture.

Of course the fetus could survive, resulting in a live birth. Also, if the mother is being monitored and an unexpected crisis occurs in her condition whereby she requires a caesarean section for her own sake, again the result is a live, preterm neonate with an abnormality. If that baby is anencephalic, the chances are that it will die fairly soon, but it could suffer in the meantime. If the baby has an abnormality that will not necessarily claim its life, then the pregnancy has been terminated, but the parents have a baby who they had decided should not live.

What if the baby has a low Apgar score and requires some resuscitation? Either you resuscitate him, resulting in a baby to be cared for, probably against the parents' wishes, although once they have seen him they might change their minds. Or you do not resuscitate him, but leave him to die, which was the original plan for the fetus. If the baby is anencephalic, perhaps the decision, in the best interests of the baby, would not be too hard to make. However, there are many other abnormalities for which termination of pregnancy is undertaken, where perhaps the decision would be ethically far more difficult for some people.

Legally, of course, there should be no dilemma. If the baby is born with any signs of life we have a duty to care for him in his own right, not as part of his parents. This does not mean that aggressive resuscitation of an anencephalic baby should be undertaken, but where the abnormality is compatible with life we are duty bound to treat the baby as we would any other (Dimond 1999, UKCC 1998). In fact, even private abortion clinics have to have neonatal resuscitation equipment available in the event of a live birth, as the *Infanticide Act 1938* states:

> ...*anyone assisting in the commission of an act, or acquiescing in an omission resulting in the death of a child born alive, may be charged with murder.*

Callahan (1995, p. 272), having highlighted the fact that some authors are antagonistic to the idea of feticide before the termination, states that she agrees that:

> *a woman's right to terminate a pregnancy does not entail or include a right to death of her fetus.*

She does believe, however, that feticide by means of intracardiac injection of potassium chloride is the right course of action. First, she believes this because it creates a safer procedure for the mother, who is entitled to the safest care possible. The description of the method of termination indicates the reason that feticide makes the process safer. Second, she believes that where a decision has been made that survival would not be in the best interests of the seriously abnormal fetus, or the child it might become, feticide is in the child's short- and long-term interests.

The Ethics Committee of the Royal College of Obstetricians and Gynaecologists (RCOG 1998, p. 11) has stated:

> *Two alternative duties ... on the paediatrician to provide care appropriate to the child's condition, or on the obstetrician to ensure that the fetus died without pain. When it comes to the borderline cases, there is, despite previous assessment, the problematic question of paediatric resuscitation if live born, leading to both intensive procedures on the neonate and the risk of extremely handicapped survival.*

According to this statement, if obstetricians are not prepared to perform feticide before the induction of labour, then a paediatrician must be present at the delivery, in order to make appropriate decisions if the need arises. Despite this statement, however, anecdotal evidence from midwives suggests that all too often fetal death is not ensured. Also, paediatricians are reluctant to attend the delivery or the baby once born, thus continuing the dilemma for the midwives. In view of the legal situation, a midwife is not at liberty to let a baby die just because the parents chose abortion, although she may feel under great pressure from them to do nothing.

The RCOG (1998, p. 17) also stated:

> *The obstetrician has a duty to protect the fetus from suffering pain in all terminations of pregnancy regardless of gestation.*
> *... For termination of pregnancy carried out at or after 24 weeks, it is therefore recommended that either feticide should be carried out ... or premedication should be given to the mother, allowing time for it to build up in the fetus.*

Many midwives have experience of babies born before 24 weeks of gestation and they would suggest that, if feticide is the right course of action from 24 weeks, then it should be a course of action carried out where abortion is conducted from 20 weeks of gestation.

Some Supervisors of Midwives feel that part of the live birth problem lies in the fact that there are so many different definitions relating to what constitutes 'signs of life'. They are quite right to point out that the wording of the definitions is different, but the principles underlying them are the same. It is also essential to remember that each practitioner is accountable for their own practice; therefore, regardless of any definition, if they believe that there are signs of life then they must act accordingly and be prepared to justify their actions or omissions.

APPLYING THE THEORIES TO ANGELA'S SITUATION

Utilitarian views

An act-utilitarian is looking to create the greatest benefit for the majority of people. In Angela's case, having the termination of pregnancy would distress Angela and Jo in the short term, and possibly in the long term. This would be balanced against: (1) their distress at losing the baby, after delivery, through natural means but possibly after him suffering; or (2) the distress at having to see him in a long-term disabled condition. Added to this could be the worry of finding quality time for their first son, so that he did not feel pushed out by his disabled brother and therefore resent him. The act-utilitarian would also consider the resource issue. Caring for a severely disabled child would be very costly in resources in its widest sense. It would be seen that very little good could come from such use of resources, whereas, by terminating the pregnancy, the resources would be available for wider use. The view of conscientious objection would probably be to uphold the right to such objection, so long as it did not stand in the way of creating all the good already determined by the decision to carry out the abortion.

Rule-utilitarians are also seeking the principle of utility, wanting the best results for the most people. However, they are more concerned with justice than act-utilitarians, so they view acts in the light of generalising a rule, rather than the specific results of the acts themselves. They would consider whether abortion for fetal abnormality, as a general rule, would create the greatest good and diminish the harm. It is quite possible that they would agree with the act-utilitarians about the abortion. However, generalising the idea of healthcare professionals having conscientious objections would result in all of them objecting to participation, thus preventing abortion for fetal abnormality that had previously been deemed a right action. They would be unlikely to uphold such views.

Deontological views

The Kantian view would consider Angela's autonomy but this would conflict with the principle of the sanctity of life. A Kantian who viewed the late gestation fetus as a person would be against killing it, not only because of the sanctity of life, but because it would be wrong for Angela to abort the fetus as a means to her own ends. By applying the principle of universalisation, a Kantian would determine whether it would be right for all women pregnant with abnormal fetuses to undergo termination of pregnancy probably deciding that it would be an immoral act to destroy all fetuses with abnormalities. Conscientious objection would be upheld as, if abortion is not desirable because of the sanctity of life, then universalisation of people refusing to participate in it would be proven to be a moral act.

A traditionalist would probably see the late gestation fetus as being a person, regardless of any disabilities, and would therefore be against the idea of abortion. By the same token, a traditionalist would be in favour of upholding the conscientious objection to participation in abortion.

A pluralist might well have a great dilemma. First, it would depend on whether the pluralist considered the late gestation fetus to be a person. If so, the pluralist's duties to Angela and those to her fetus would conflict. The pluralist may consider that to allow the fetus to be born and then suffer was not beneficent, non-maleficent or just. On the other hand, the pluralist may decide that feticide did not fulfil their duties either. The duties to Angela would not include consideration of how she would cope with a disabled baby, as the pluralist would not consider the consequences of actions, only the rightness. It is probable that the termination of pregnancy, would not be sanctioned. The pluralist's duties to those with conscientious objections would suggest that their views should be upheld, as to disregard them would be seen as a breach of beneficence, non-maleficence, justice and probably fidelity.

REFERENCES

Andrews G (ed) 1997 Women's sexual health. Baillière Tindall, London
Bruner J 1999 Born twice. BBC TV, 20 October
Burnard P, Chapman C M 1993 Professional and ethical issues in nursing, 2nd edn. Scutari, Harrow

Callahan J C 1995 Ensuring a stillborn: the ethics of lethal injection in late abortion. In: Callahan J C (ed) Reproduction, ethics, and the law. Feminist perspectives, Introduction to Part III. Indiana University, Indianapolis

Cuckle H S, Wald N J 1984 Introduction: In: Wald N J (ed) Antenatal and neonatal screening. Oxford University Press, Oxford

Dimond B 1999 A legal right to abortion: right or wrong? British Journal of Midwifery 7(6):355–357

Jones S R 1999 Conscientious objection to participation in abortion. British Journal of Midwifery 7(11):677–679

Mahowald M B 1995 As if there were fetuses without women: a remedial essay. In: Callahan J C (ed) Reproduction, ethics, and the law. Feminist perspectives. Indiana University, Indianapolis

Morgan D, Lee R G 1991 Blackstone's guide to the Human Fertilisation and Embryology Act 1990. Blackstone, London

Noonan J T 1999 How to argue about abortion. In: Palmer M (ed) Moral problems in medicine. Lutterworth, Cambridge

Palmer M 1999 Moral problems in medicine. Lutterworth Cambridge

Purdy L, Tooley M 1999 Is abortion murder? In: Palmer M (ed) Moral problems in medicine. Lutterworth, Cambridge

Richards M P M 1988 Social and ethical problems of fetal diagnosis and screening. Journal of Reproductive Infant Psychology 7:171–185

Royal College of Midwives 1997 Conscientious objection. Position paper 17. RCM, London

Royal College of Obstetricians and Gynaecologists 1998 A consideration of the law and ethics in relation to late termination of pregnancy for fetal abnormality. RCOG, London

Royal College of Paediatrics and Child Health 1997 Withholding or withdrawing treatment in children. A framework for practice. RCPCH, London

UKCC 1992 Code of professional conduct. for the nurse, midwife and health visitor. UKCC, London

UKCC 1996 Guidelines for professional practice. UKCC, London

UKCC 1998 Midwives rules and code of practice. UKCC, London

Warnock M 1998 An intelligent person's guide to ethics. Duckworth, London

SUGGESTED ADDITIONAL READING

Caplan A 1995 Wrongful-birth lawsuits are wrong solution. In: Caplan A. Moral matters. John Wiley, Chichester, p 17

Drazek M 1999 Termination of pregnancy: why are live births occurring? British Journal of Midwifery 7(12):742–748

Fox M 1998 A woman's right to choose? A feminist critique. In: Harris J, Holm S (eds) The future of human reproduction. Clarendon, Oxford, ch 5, p 77

Gans Epner J E, Jonas H S, Seckinger D L 1998 Late-term abortion. Journal of the American Medical Association 280(8):724–729

Grimes D A 1998 Late-term abortion. Journal of the American Medical Association 280(8):747

Herring J 1997 Children's abortion rights. In: Kennedy I, Grubb A (eds) Medical Law Review 5(3):257–268

Holt J 1996 Screening and the perfect baby. In: Frith L (ed) Ethics and midwifery. Issues in contemporary practice. Butterworth Heinemann, Oxford, p 140

Kenny M 1986 Abortion. The whole story. Quartet Books, London

Marquis D 1997 An argument that abortion is wrong. In: LaFollette H (ed) Ethics in practice. An anthology. Blackwell, Oxford, ch 7, p 91

Rothman B K 1997 Redefining abortion. In: LaFollette H (ed) Ethics in practice. An anthology. Blackwell, Oxford, ch 8, p 103

Thomson J J 1997 A defense of abortion. In: LaFollette H (ed) Ethics in practice. An anthology. Blackwell, Oxford, ch 5, p 69

Warren M A 1997 On the moral and legal status of abortion. In: LaFollette H (ed) Ethics in practice. An anthology. Blackwell, Oxford, ch 6, p 79

Whitfield A 1993 Common law duties to unborn children. In: Kennedy I, Grubb A (eds) Medical Law Review 1(1):28–52

9

Assisted conception – a right or a dilemma?

Claire is an experienced community midwife, having worked with the same group of general practitioners (GPs), within a set geographical area, for the last nine years. She thought that she had experienced most situations that can unexpectedly happen to a midwife – until recently.

Claire had visited Gina at home in order to undertake a booking interview. She discovered that Gina had one child, born five years ago in another part of the country. She also discovered that the current pregnancy was the result of assisted conception, although Gina would not be drawn on any further discussion of the matter. Gina wanted to have the baby in the local obstetric unit but she wanted an early discharge after the delivery. After further discussion it was agreed that Gina could have a DOMINO (domestic in and out) booking, with minimal visits to the hospital.

Gina attended routine visits with Claire. At each visit she was accompanied by a friend, Estelle, who always had questions to ask and at whom Gina always looked before making decisions. Such questions related to the screening tests, which were offered and accepted, and parentcraft classes, which were declined. As the pregnancy progressed, Claire started to feel that there was something different about Gina and Estelle. She began to wonder whether they were a lesbian couple and the assisted conception had been donor insemination. She did not like to ask and she kept her thoughts to herself.

At 36 weeks of gestation, Claire talked to Gina about preparation for labour; she asked if Estelle would be her birth partner. After a long, uncomfortable pause, Gina stated that Estelle and Estelle's husband Marcus would both be present for the labour and delivery, as she was the host surrogate mother for their baby. They had had in-vitro fertilisation (IVF) of their own gametes and the two resulting embryos had been transferred to Gina, although only one embryo implanted successfully. They had wanted to keep their situation as quiet as possible. Claire was a little stunned, having had no experience of such a situation before, but she tried to appear fairly nonchalant and accepting of the information.

The next day Claire looked for a Trust policy on dealing with surrogacy, but she could not find one. She sought the assistance of her Supervisor of Midwives and discussed her anxieties about the documentation after delivery, also what to do to prevent difficulties if Gina changed her mind after the baby was born. It was agreed that the mother's details would be used in the documentation and they would deal with any change of plans if and when they occurred.

At 39 weeks and two days, Gina's labour commenced during the night and she contacted Claire. Gina was taken into hospital by Steve, her husband, who remained in the visitors' waiting room throughout the labour and delivery. Claire was at the hospital waiting for Gina, hoping for a few minutes alone with her before the commissioning parents arrived. Claire ascertained that, initially, Gina had been happy to agree to Estelle and Marcus being present for the labour and delivery. However, as the pregnancy had progressed, she felt that Estelle's natural excitement had caused her to become demanding and dictatorial. Gina was worried that this attitude might affect her ability to relax and that, as Estelle did not want Gina to have any invasive methods of pain relief in case they affected the baby, this would be very important. Claire said that she would do whatever she could to help Gina and that she would try to pick up on any non-verbal cues.

When Estelle and Marcus arrived they seemed very caring and supportive of Gina. Claire made it clear that there would be times when she would ask them to leave, such as during any intimate examinations or if Gina needed to use a bedpan. They accepted Claire's decision. The labour progressed well with Gina using Entonox when required. When the second stage of labour was reached, Estelle stated that the baby was to be given directly to her after delivery. Claire looked at Gina's facial expression but said nothing.

The baby girl was born in good condition, on to the bed. When Claire had cut the cord she wrapped the baby in the prepared towel and handed her to Gina, while congratulating everyone. Estelle said nothing but the atmosphere in the room became tense. Gina held the baby close, smiled at her, kissed her cheek then held her out to Estelle.

QUESTIONS FOR CONSIDERATION BY THE READER

1. Is surrogacy legal in the UK?
2. The documentation was to be completed with 'the mother's details', but who was the mother in this situation?
3. Did Claire act correctly in ignoring Estelle's instructions?
4. What should Claire have done if Gina had refused to continue with the surrogacy arrangements once the baby was born?

QUESTION 1: IS SURROGACY LEGAL IN THE UK?

Surrogacy has been legal in the UK since July 1985 when the *Surrogacy Arrangements Act 1985* came into force. This Act was then amended by the *Human Fertilisation and Embryology Act 1990 (HFE Act 1990)*. In June 1997 the Brazier committee was set up to reconsider surrogacy, particularly with regard to the apparent circumvention of the law with regard to payment. Neither the original nor the amended Act dealt with the financial issues, assuming that the *Adoption Act 1976* would deter people from entering into financial agreements, as this Act forbids the effective buying of babies (Freeman 1999). In some cases the law pertaining to adoption probably was effective, but not all surrogacy cases result in adoption, therefore not all cases are protected. Also, where it would be acceptable for reasonable expenses to be paid, some people were thought to be somewhat creative with their assessment of expenses and in their methods of paying them. The Brazier Report (Department of Health 1998a) recommended that there should be a new Surrogacy Act which bans payments other than statutorily defined expenses, requires surrogacy agencies to be registered and enforces a code of practice. However, Linda Nelson, who replaced Kim Cotton as chairperson of the organisation Childlessness Overcome Through Surrogacy (COTS), believes that banning payments would be wrong. She feels that a payment of £10 000 is reasonable recompense for the time and trouble expended by surrogate mothers (Mercer 1999).

While there are a number of means of obtaining a surrogate pregnancy, there are two overall types of surrogacy. There is 'straight surrogacy' in which the surrogate's own ovum is fertilised by the intended father's sperm, by artificial insemination or, indeed, by sexual intercourse. The second type is 'host IVF surrogacy', where the embryo is created by using the commissioning couple's gametes, or donated gametes, then transferring the embryo to the surrogate's uterus (Cotton 1999). The first type may require little or no outside assistance, whereas the second type obviously requires the assistance of a licensed clinic. In the USA the two types of surrogacy are defined as 'traditional' and 'gestational' respectively, but laws vary from state to state (Z 1999).

QUESTION 2: THE DOCUMENTATION WAS TO BE COMPLETED WITH 'THE MOTHER'S DETAILS', BUT WHO WAS THE MOTHER IN THIS SITUATION?

It is understandable that there could be confusion as to who is the mother in this case. On the one hand there is the fact that the embryo has implanted in Gina; her body has nurtured it, she has experienced all the systematic changes inherent in pregnancy and she has undergone labour and delivery. She may also have experienced some psychological changes or anxieties during this process (Smith 1998). On the other hand, the genetic make-up of the baby comes from Estelle and Marcus, and the whole process has been undertaken in order to provide them with this baby. The UK law is clear as to the definition of 'mother' in cases of assisted conception (*HFE Act 1990*, Section 27 (1)):

> *The woman who is carrying or has carried a child as a result*
> *of the placing in her of an embryo or of sperm and eggs,*
> *and no other woman, is to be treated as the mother of the*
> *child.*

This position is contrary to that in California (which differs from some other States in the USA), where the gamete suppliers are deemed the parents in surrogacy cases (Caplan 1995).

Subsection (2) of section 27 includes the fact that an adoption order withdraws the rights and responsibilities of the mother as defined above, thus allowing parental rights to be transferred to the adoptive parents.

Section 28 of the *HFE Act 1990* defines the term 'father' in cases of assisted conception:

If –

(a) at the time of the placing in her of the embryo or of sperm and eggs or of her artificial insemination, the woman was party to a marriage, and

(b) the creation of the embryo carried by her was not brought about with the sperm of the other party to the marriage,

then ... the other party to the marriage shall be treated as the father of the child unless it is shown that he did not consent to the placing in her of the embryo or the sperm and eggs or to her insemination (as the case may be).

At the time of birth of the baby in this case, Gina is the '*mother*' and Steve is the '*father*' – if he accepted her surrogate role. If Steve was not a consenting party to the surrogacy then the 'father' would be deemed to be unknown, even though the genetic father was in fact known to be Marcus. In effect, Marcus' sperm was donated and giving the parental rights inherent in the legal term of 'father' to a sperm donor could create dilemmas. For instance, in general, determining that the donor is the father would remove his right to anonymity (Deech 1999a) and bestow rights and responsibilities not in keeping with his initial intention. In this particular case, although Marcus wants the rights and responsibilities, giving him equal parental rights could infringe the rights of the legal mother, Gina, as they are not married to each other nor in a common law relationship.

The law is quite clear, therefore, that the midwife must complete the documentation, including the birth notification, with the surrogate's details. The baby will be registered by Gina and, as she has the genetic make-up of at least one of the commissioning couple, then Estelle and Marcus can make an application for a 'parental order' within six months of the baby's birth; they will not need to apply for adoption. In order to do this, the baby must be living with them in the UK, Channel Islands or Isle of Man (*HFE Act 1990,* section 30) and Gina and Steve must have consented to the arrangement.

QUESTION 3: DID CLAIRE ACT CORRECTLY IN IGNORING ESTELLE'S INSTRUCTIONS?

Although the legal position is clear, the ethical situation may have felt very unclear to Claire. She was obviously aware of her duty towards Gina as a childbearing woman, albeit that Gina's intentions, at least at the outset of the pregnancy, were to relinquish the baby. Claire had to treat her as an autonomous woman with regard to her care in labour and with regard to her decisions once the baby was born (see Ch. 7 on Autonomy and consent). She had to act in accordance with Gina's needs and requests, as with any other pregnant woman (English & Sommerville 1996).

It would be understandable for Claire to have wondered what, if any, her duties were to Estelle and Marcus. They were, after all, the intended parents. She could well have wondered whether she should encourage a relationship between them and the baby as soon as she was born, particularly for Estelle, who would not have experienced what most women do in carrying and delivering a baby. If all went to plan they would be starting their roles and activities as parents as soon as possible; therefore, creating a good start from birth could be seen to be very important. In fact, apart from the usual duty of care with regard to health and safety in that part of the hospital, plus the usual level of care afforded to birth partners or companions, Claire had no extra duty of care until Gina had consented to them taking the baby.

Claire picked up on the verbal and non-verbal cues from Gina and acted accordingly, thus upholding autonomy and providing advocacy for her (UKCC 1996). She did not try to stay outside the situation by ignoring the non-verbal communication and just obeying the verbal commands. Once Gina had passed the baby to Estelle and Marcus, with a view to them adopting the roles of parents, then Claire would be free to undertake the activities of a midwife with regard to the care of a new baby and development of good parent–baby interaction. This would obviously need to be undertaken with great sensitivity towards Gina.

QUESTION 4: WHAT SHOULD CLAIRE HAVE DONE IF GINA HAD REFUSED TO CONTINUE WITH THE SURROGACY ARRANGEMENTS ONCE THE BABY WAS BORN?

The *Surrogacy Arrangements Act 1985* was amended by the *HFE Act 1990* to incorporate the fact that:

> *No surrogacy arrangement is enforceable by or against any of the persons making it. (section 1A)*

This means that Gina could legally decide to keep the baby, and Estelle and Marcus could also decide that they did not want the baby after all. As statutory law allows for both parties to change their minds, claims of breach of contract would be futile.

Claire's first action would have to have been to protect Gina and the baby, emotionally and possibly physically, by removing Estelle and Marcus from the room. Probably she would then have wanted to support Estelle and Marcus; therefore, escorting them from the room and accompanying them to a private area could achieve both objectives initially. It may be that Gina would want to be supported by Steve, thus giving Claire the opportunity to deal with Estelle and Marcus herself or get someone else to help. Having dispatched someone to get a drink for the couple, Claire could enlist the help of the manager, who would need to know what had happened anyway. She could also seek help from a Supervisor of Midwives, who could support Claire as well as the couple; the hospital chaplain, if the couple felt that this would help them; or the bereavement midwife/officer might have some idea of how to support these people who are suffering their own sense of loss. As this is not an adoptive situation, there is unlikely to be a social worker involved and, while they have expertise that might help, not every couple would readily accept the involvement of social workers.

The Brazier Report (Department of Health 1998b) suggests that this traumatic situation occurs in only an estimated 4–5% of surrogacy arrangements, but it results in devastation for the commissioning couple. Also the surrogate has a baby that was unplanned as far as her family organisation is concerned. In Gina's case, her son would not have been prepared for the sister who is about to share his life, in the way that most parents prepare their children. On the other hand, how does an existing child cope when its mother has a baby and effectively gives it away? It is possible that some children will understand and accept the explanation given by the parents without trauma, but perhaps not all.

FURTHER DISCUSSION

According to Deech (1999b) one in six couples suffer infertility. These figures are determined by the uptake of fertility investigation and treatment; it is therefore uncertain how accurate they are as some couples may not seek assistance. It could be argued that a proportion of those who choose, from the outset, not to have children may be infertile without any awareness of it, but this is irrelevant in this situation, as surely it is the frustrated desire to have children that is in question. Infertility is often seen as a female issue, despite the fact that men also desire to have children. Also, while this chapter considers infertility and the treatment of it, it is accepted that not every woman will want children. Berg (1995, p. 80) acknowledges this but notes that childless women often have to live with others' perceptions of them as selfish. However, for those who are thwarted in their intended achievement of parenthood, it is important to recognise that availability of infertility treatment is as important as the provision of contraception and abortion services for fertile women.

Ethical issues in assisted reproductive techniques generally

Do people have a right to have a child?

In 1976, Mrs Justice Heilbron, in 'Re D', declared that sterilisation of an 11-year-old girl with Soto's syndrome, which causes early sexual maturity, would infringe her basic human right to bear a child once she was of an age for self-determination (Brazier 1998, p. 66). Also, Article 12 of the European Convention for the Protection of Human Rights and Fundamental Freedoms states (Wadham & Mountfield 1999):

> *Men and women of marriageable age have the right to marry and to found a family, according to the national laws governing the exercise of this right.*

These statements suggest that a legal right exists, but what is a 'right'? According to Warnock (1998):

> *A right is something you claim, and which you can properly prevent other people from infringing. It is an area of freedom for an individual which someone else must allow him to exercise, as a matter of justice.*

With this definition in mind, it seems inappropriate to claim that people have a right to have a child, as this would place an impossible burden on outside agencies to ensure that all those who claimed the right achieved it. It could depend, however, on how we define a 'child'. It could be possible to ensure that everyone has *one* child if all the children who are in institutions were placed with people who wanted children. However, most people appear to want babies, preferably born to them with their own genetic make-up (Berg 1995, p. 80). If they cannot achieve this naturally or with assistance, then some are prepared to accept donated gametes, or a host surrogate, or both.

Perhaps it would be more correct to suggest that everyone has the right to try to have a child. This creates less of a burden on those working in assisted conception to achieve success every time. If we consider that people do have the right to try to have a child, then this means all people – and that would include single women and single men, despite the sexual persuasion of either sex, plus post-menopausal women. Judging by the public debate which is evident whenever the media indicate that there has been such an occurrence, it could be suggested that many individuals would not be in favour of this practice (whether the person is homosexual or not). In fact, the debate in the House of Lords regarding the outlawing of treatment for single women was lost by only one vote (Brazier 1998). However, formulating conditions suggests that not everyone should have that right; therefore this could be deemed to be discriminatory practice. The *Human Rights Act 1998* appears only to consider such rights as pertaining to married couples and Montgomery (1997, p. 393) states that English law has not considered 'the right to have a child as being a matter of individual entitlement'.

If it is considered that people have the right to try to have a child, by natural or assisted means, then funding would have to be found for those who could not afford the treatment. Funding the less fortunate in society could also be deemed discriminatory practice, but it is unlikely to happen. It is probable that society in general would not choose to spend limited resources on infertility treatment at the expense of immunisation and screening programmes, or free prescriptions for children, the elderly and certain other disadvantaged groups in society. The National Health Service purse is not bottomless. In order to be free from claims of bias or discrimination, perhaps it would be reasonable for health authorities to provide the basic requirements for all patients/clients in the first instance, followed by the more common 'extras'; this would be an objective view. Subjectively, however, the high-powered and expensive treatments feel like the basics when it concerns ourselves and our families.

There is also the question of whether it is right to interfere with nature in this way. It could be argued that healthcare professionals interfere with nature every day: we immunise against disease, fight infection, put fluoride in the water and undertake surgical procedures, generally with little complaint from the public; rather, there is usually an expectation of more. However, where procreation and the use of genetic material is concerned, some people are less accepting of the interference. The Roman Catholic Church is just one of the religions that condemn most of the invasive fertility interventions. It is particularly against the methods that include fertilisation outside the woman's body, or use of donor gametes. This rules out IVF and any donor situation, such as donor insemination, despite the belief that it is the duty of married Roman Catholic couples to produce families. In particular, artificial insemination by donor is considered equivalent to adultery.

One area that creates major debate is that of producing 'designer babies', and whether this is the start of yet another slippery slope towards eugenics. Concern is fuelled by the setting up of a sperm bank for the breeding of superbabies: the Repository for Germinal Choice, in California (Caplan 1995). In addition to this, the Internet offers ova from fashion models (Lowther & Fraser 1999), which suggests that we could aim for a future generation of people who have both brains and beauty – although it seems unbelievable that models would wish to put themselves through the discomfort and inconvenience of stimulated ovulation, unless they are out of work.

This, in itself, might suggest something less than the perfection being sought and that is before the random mix of genes.

At one time couples either came to terms with not 'being blessed' with children, or they could fulfil their need for children by adoption. Unfortunately, for those who would be interested, there are currently very few babies for adoption, which also creates the problem of very tight criteria being set for approval of would-be adopters, making it an unrealistic option for most couples. Another option could be to attempt to correct the mental morbidity, not by assisting with reproduction, but by assisting people to come to terms with childlessness. There is a support group where help and guidance can be sought – the National Association for the Childless – and there are many couples who have adjusted their life plans accordingly.

Ethical concerns regarding various methods of assisted reproductive technology

It is accepted that some people are against assisted conception of any kind; therefore, the concerns dealt with here will be those where people do not start with this antipathetic view.

Ovulatory stimulation

Where the intention is to stimulate the maturation of one follicle, there would generally be no objections. However, where hyperstimulation is concerned, some people would worry with regard to the physiological effect on the woman's ovaries and, therefore, her morbidity. In addition to this possible problem, there are concerns regarding the possibility of multiple pregnancy, particularly where more than two embryos are transferred to the woman's uterus, or more than two ova and sperm are transferred to the fallopian tube(s) (see the paragraph after GIFT, ZIFT and IVF).

Intrauterine insemination

Where this is with the partner's sperm there is generally no ethical concern. However, if the technique was used in conjunction with hyperstimulation of the ovaries, then the concern regarding multiple pregnancy would be relevant.

Gamete intra-fallopian transfer (GIFT)

In this technique ova and sperm are transferred, separated by an air bubble, into one or both of the fallopian tubes. The intention is that fertilisation will take place inside the woman's body, for this reason: religions that are opposed to many of the assisted reproductive techniques appear to accept this technique. Multiple pregnancy and the potential problems are also concerns.

Zygote intra-fallopian transfer (ZIFT)

A major concern here is the fact that fertilisation takes place outside the body, then the zygote(s) is placed into the fallopian tube, which is seen as more than just assisting nature. The Roman Catholic Church is against this procedure for that reason. Multiple pregnancy and the potential problems are also concerns.

In vitro fertilisation (IVF) and embryo transfer (ET)

This involves fertilisation outside the body, then transfer of the embryo(s) to the woman's uterus. Objections are similar to those expressed regarding ZIFT. Multiple pregnancy and the potential problems are also concerns.

While multiple pregnancy may solve some of the problems for people with fertility problems, there is the risk of increased perinatal mortality and morbidity. Added to the natural distress created by death, disease or abnormality, there is the problem that the maternity and neonatal units may not be equipped to cope. The possibility of multiple pregnancy in itself raises important ethical issues. It is thought that multiple pregnancy gives rise to greater risk of fetal abnormality (Bergh et al 1999, Challoner 1999), and those for whom conception is considered to be the beginning of life find this practice of creating abnormality unacceptable, especially if destruction of the fetus(es) is the end result.

Pregnancies that are conceived naturally, as opposed to technologically, are most commonly the result of fertilisation of a single ovum, produced during the ovulatory phase of the human menstrual cycle. High-order multiples in spontaneous pregnancy is rare (Challoner 1999). In both IVF and GIFT/ZIFT superovulation is stimulated by drug therapy; ova retrieval then takes place at the expected time of ovulation. In the case of IVF, fertilisation takes place in vitro in the laboratory. At one time, where five or six ova were successfully fertilised, they were all returned to the woman's uterus. However, doctors performing IVF are no longer at liberty to transfer more than three embryos or ova and sperm (HFEA 1998a). In fact, the British Fertility Society has recommended that no more than two embryos should be transferred (HFEA 1998a); the tone and language of the seventh Annual Report appears to support this view (HFEA 1998b).

Where GIFT is used, as explained previously, the ova and sperm are placed in the fallopian tube(s) where fertilisation would normally occur, in vivo. Practitioners who use this method of treatment are not directed regarding the number of ova replaced. The *Human Fertilisation and Embryology Act 1990*, while formalising the licensing authority in respect of IVF and research, did not encompass GIFT (Brazier 1998). Many professionals feel that this was an unfortunate omission, as there have been reports of some specialists transferring four or more ova at one time (Vines 1990). In fact, according to Manning (1990), one particular practitioner who was opposed to limiting the numbers is reported to have recorded, in a professional journal, his transfer of 11 or more. In order to prevent some of the disasters of high-order multiple pregnancy, some consultants advocate selective reduction of the number of fetuses. This is generally carried out by injection of potassium chloride into the gestational sacs of those easiest to reach, with the aid of ultrasound scanning. Those who are against abortion may well be against this process too, although Muslims will allow it if the viability of the pregnancy is very low, or if the mother's life is in danger (Serour 1998, p. 191).

The reason for transferring more than one or two embryos, or ova and sperm, was understandable: the doctors were concerned with giving that woman, or couple, the best possible chance of having a baby at the end of the process – one that is long and expensive (physically, emotionally, socially and financially). If, however, events have shown this to be unwise, then surely doctors should resist the practice. If such high-order multiple conceptions occur, then the pregnancy itself is at risk. The live births that follow successful multiple pregnancy are high-risk babies, often preterm with increased rates of morbidity and mortality. It could be argued that there is a duty to maintain those babies already conceived, and those delivered, rather than expend financial and human resources on expensive, possibly vain, attempts to alleviate the problems of infertile people.

Intracytoplasmic sperm injection (ICSI)

This technique, developed from a fortuitous accident, is now widely used in cases of male infertility, but the resulting children are to be followed to determine any abnormalities. It may or may not be used following sperm aspiration, which can be achieved in a number of ways: from the epididymus microsurgically (microsurgical epididymal sperm aspiration; MESA) or percutaneously (percutaneous epididymal sperm aspiration; PESA), or from testicular tissue (testicular sperm aspiration; TESA). The major concerns are that sperm that would not manage to fertilise an egg in normal circumstances may pass on chromosomal abnormalities. In particular, it is thought that where a man's infertility is due to genetic abnormality, this may be recreated in his son (Challoner 1999). Also, research in Australia suggests significant evidence of mild delays in development at one year, compared with children conceived naturally (Challoner 1999, HFEA 1998b). Some people believe that it is immoral to create a problem for the child by way of fulfilling the parents' needs. It appears that we are back to Kant's view regarding treating others as a means to our own ends.

Donor gametes

While many people have no objection to assisted conception using the gametes of the couple involved, they draw the line at use of donated gametes. For Roman Catholics and Muslims (Serour 1998) this is, in effect, similar to adultery. Another aspect of concern is the anonymity of donors. For some people anonymity is very important and it is thought that they would discontinue donation if anonymity were no longer assured. However, there are also many people who think that the persons created, once of adult years, should have access to the information of their origins. The stance on this issue, as with many others, varies throughout Europe. In Scandinavia, for instance, Denmark upholds anonymity, while in Norway and Sweden anonymity has been abandoned. In Sweden, they found that the number of young donors (usually medical students) reduced, but they have been replaced by older men (Nielsen 1999).

Surrogacy

Surrogacy can take many forms. The surrogate may use her own ovum with sperm from either the commissioning man or a donor, or she may be a complete host. This would entail implantation of donated gametes or embryos, the donors being either the commissioning couple, other donors or a mixture of the two. This is possibly the most controversial of the assisted reproductive techniques, and is not accepted by some religions, notably Roman Catholics and Muslims. One reason for public debate regarding this issue relates to the tug-of-love babies who hit the headlines in the USA, the UK (Challoner 1999) and Australia (Otlowski 1999), some of which included contracts and financial payments. As always, the public appear to be divided. Some people believe that a bargain should be honoured, particularly if the baby is genetically that of the commissioning couple, while others cannot understand the morality of a woman bearing a child and then giving it away. It could be argued that this is no different from adoption, where a woman bears a child then allows it to be given to others. However, some people have always held the belief that adoption is wrong, for the same reasons as surrogacy. Others would say that they can accept adoption because, usually, the mother did not intend to become pregnant, whereas in surrogacy the pregnancy and handover is planned.

Tong (1995) examined a number of models of surrogacy arrangement to see which would be the most appropriate to benefit women as a whole. She narrowed her choice down to two: a contract model and an adoption model, before settling on the adoption model as being the least heartless.

Embryo research

It could be said that where there is IVF there is embryo research, and to a certain extent that cannot be argued against. Even if a formal programme of experimentation and research is not in operation, records must be kept accurately and audits undertaken, thereby giving an ongoing picture and creating the mechanism for retrospective studies. The issue of research and experimentation continues to be debated, particularly with regard to gene therapy and cloning. This debate will not be continued here, other than to allow a moment to contemplate the future.

If scientists eventually manage to eradicate genetic disease by gene therapy, they will undoubtedly turn to the problems of environmental factors in their search for beneficent perfection – not looking to create a specific genetic mould for malignant reasons. To remove environmental anomalies, the scientists will probably further develop the idea of ectogenesis. As this facility increases, the demand for midwives will disappear, while the need for technicians will increase. One wonders what the midwifery education curriculum will look like in the interim years.

APPLYING THE THEORIES TO CLAIRE'S ACTIONS

Utilitarian views

One of the major problems with utilitarianism is the fact that consequences need to be predicted before action is taken: where human behaviour is concerned, particularly when emotion is likely to be a key component, it can be difficult to predict likely outcomes. In the case in question, everyone seemed to get what they wanted, which would suggest a good action from both the act-utilitarian and rule-utilitarian perspectives. However, if Claire could have known for sure that the end result would be as it was, then she would have been on safer ground and her actions would have been more appropriate. In effect, her actions were a gamble. She presumed that she had read Gina's non-verbal communication correctly, although, if she had got it wrong, she could have caused distress to Gina. She could also have received an angry response from Estelle, for not obeying her instructions. Whether or not Estelle had any rights, creating antagonism in the delivery room would not have been good for anybody. It would have been preferable to ask Gina what she wanted, then there would have been more certainty regarding the outcome.

Deontological views

Ignoring the fact that a Kantian would probably view surrogacy as immoral, as it would not stand up to the test of universalisation, the Kantian would be concerned that Claire should not treat Gina as a means to Estelle's ends. Therefore, Claire was right to consider Gina's perceived needs as paramount. If Claire had misinterpreted Gina's facial expression, resulting in upsetting her, then this would have been unfortunate, but not wrong as her intentions were good.

A traditionalist would probably be against the notion of surrogacy and would support Claire's actions; however, an advocate of this perspective would then prefer that Gina did not give the baby to Estelle.

A pluralist would deem that Claire should do what was best for Gina, to whom she had a duty of care. She should ensure that her actions were just, that they would be good for her and do no harm. She would also be expected to keep her promise to be Gina's advocate, based on non-verbal cues, which she did. A pluralist, then, would probably applaud Claire's actions as they would not be concerned regarding possible consequences.

REFERENCES

Berg B J 1995 Listening to the voices of the infertile. In: Callahan J C (ed) Reproduction, ethics and the law. Feminist perspectives. Indiana University, Indianapolis

Bergh T, Ericson A, Hillensjö T, Nygren K-G, Wennerholm U-B 1999 Deliveries and children born after in-vitro fertilisation in Sweden 1982–95: a retrospective cohort study. Lancet 354: 1579–1585

Brazier M 1998 Reproductive rights: feminism or patriarchy. In: Harris J, Holm S (eds) The future of human reproduction. Clarendon, Oxford

Caplan A 1995 Moral matters. John Wiley, Chichester

Challoner J 1999 The baby makers. The history of artificial conception. Channel 4 Books, Oxford

Cotton K 1999 What is surrogacy? Available at: http://www.surrogacy.org.uk/whatis.htm

Deech R 1999a Family law and genetics. In: Brownsword R, Cornish W R, Llewelyn M (eds) Law and human genetics. Regulating a revolution. Hart Publishing, Oxford, p 105

Deech R 1999b Welcome to the HFEA website: chairman's welcome. Available at: http://www.hfea.gov.uk

Department of Health 1998a Surrogacy – review for health ministers of current arrangements for payments and regulation (Brazier Report) – executive summary. HMSO, London

Department of Health 1998b Surrogacy – review for health ministers of current arrangements for payments and regulation (Brazier Report). HMSO, London

English V, Sommerville A 1996 Mothers in law. Health Service Journal 16 May:6

Freeman M 1999 Does surrogacy have a future after Brazier? Medical Law Review 7:3

Human Fertilisation and Embryology Authority 1998a Code of practice, 4th edn. HFEA, London

Human Fertilisation and Embryology Authority 1998b Seventh annual report. HFEA, London

Lowther W, Fraser L 1999 Models auction their eggs on the Internet for $150 000. The Mail on Sunday 24 October: 5

Manning M 1990 The painful gamete intra-fallopian transfer of life? New Statesman and Society 11 May:12–15

Mercer A 1999 End of the line. Nursery World 18 November: 10–11

Montgomery J 1997 Health care law. Oxford University Press, Oxford

Nielsen L 1999 Genetics, the family and human rights (Scandinavian perspective). Presentation at international conference on biomedicine, the family and human rights, Oxford, UK, August 1999

Otlowski M 1999 Reflections on Australia's first litigated surrogacy case. Medical Law Review 7:38–57

Re D (a minor) (wardship: sterilisation) 1976 1 All England Reports 326

Serour G I 1998 Reproductive choice: a Muslim perspective. In: Harris J, Holm S (eds) The future of human reproduction. Clarendon, Oxford

Smith M 1998 Maternal–fetal attachment in surrogate mothers. British Journal of Midwifery. 6(3):188–192

Tong R 1995 Feminist perspectives and gestational motherhood: the search for a unified legal focus. In: Callahan J C (ed) Reproduction, ethics and the law. Feminist perspectives. Indiana University, Indianapolis

UKCC 1996 Guidelines for professional practice. UKCC, London

Vines G 1990 Doctors warn of loophole in embryology bill. New Scientist 31 March:21

Wadham J, Mountfield H 1999 Blackstone's guide to the Human Rights Act 1998. Blackstone, London

Warnock M 1998 An intelligent person's guide to ethics. Gerald Duckworth, London

Z J 1999 Definition and types of surrogacy. Available at: http://www.surromomsonline.com/articles/define.htm

SUGGESTED ADDITIONAL READING.

Adams A E 1994 Reproducing the womb. Images of childbirth in science, feminist theory, and literature. Cornell University, Ithaca, NY

Berer M (ed) 1999 Living without children. Reproductive Health Matters 7(13) May 1999 [various articles]

Bowden P 1997 Mothering. In: Caring. Gender sensitive ethics. Routledge, London, ch 1, p 21

British Medical Association 1998 Human genetics. Choice and responsibility. Oxford University Press, Oxford

Caplan A 1995 Moral matters. John Wiley, Chichester

Drewett R 1994 Uncertain comforts: the justification for treating infertility. Journal of Reproductive and Infant Psychology 12:173–178

Frith L 1996 Reproductive technologies and midwifery. In: Frith L (ed) Ethics and midwifery. Issues in contemporary practice. Butterworth Heinemann, Oxford, ch 10, p 170

Lavery S, Trew G 1998 Assisted conception: ethics and advances. Gynaecology Update 4 February: 212–221

Neville K 1998 Mind matters. Nursing Times 94(41):40–41

10

Withholding or withdrawing treatment

Jasmine is 16 days old and is currently cared for in an incubator in a neonatal unit (NNU) about 10 miles from her parents' home. She was born at 30 weeks of gestation following a fairly rapid spontaneous preterm labour, for which there was no apparent reason. At delivery her Apgar scores were poor and she has been ventilated ever since. Ultrasound scans have shown intraventricular haemorrhages which have dilated the ventricles and significant areas of brain damage. Two neonatologists have reviewed Jasmine's case and both are very concerned regarding her prognosis.

Christina is one of the midwives who has been caring for Jasmine regularly since her admission to the NNU. As she conducts the handover to a member of the night staff, she reflects on the tiring shift that has just come to an end. It had been an upsetting day. As usual, she had talked to Jasmine every time she had attended to her and, as usual, there was no response to touch or sound. There had been two episodes of convulsions, which had been increasing in frequency and duration over the past few days. Following the later episode, and the review by the second doctor, Jasmine's parents had become very distressed and their once positive outlook seemed to have deserted them. Christina found it very difficult to encourage them while not building false hopes.

As she collected her belongings from her locker and started the long walk to the car park, Christina contemplated the ordeal to be faced the next morning. There was to be a case conference, led by the consultant neonatologist in charge of Jasmine's case – initially without the parents present – to consider the way forward with her care. This would be Christina's first experience of such a discussion. When on her own, Christina could argue for both continuation and discontinuation of treatment: she could see at least two points of view. But how would she cope when asked to express her views within the group? Most of the others who were involved with Jasmine's care had more experience than Christina; all she felt that she had was an opinion. Although she could contemplate two sides of the argument, she also had an inbuilt feeling that supported one of these views. She wondered how appropriate it would be to explain this at the meeting.

Christina reached her car and consciously had to transfer her thoughts to her driving, but she felt that she would have a troubled night, despite her tiredness.

QUESTIONS FOR CONSIDERATION BY THE READER:

1. Should Christina be worried about expressing her opinion at the case conference?
2. Can treatment be withheld or withdrawn from Jasmine?
3. With whom does the final decision rest?

QUESTION 1: SHOULD CHRISTINA BE WORRIED ABOUT EXPRESSING HER OPINION AT THE CASE CONFERENCE?

It is understandable that Christina feels anxious about the planned case conference, particularly as she has no previous experience upon which to reflect. This meeting of professionals involved in Jasmine's care will have serious implications for her. There could be a decision to stop treatment, with the ultimate outcome being Jasmine's death; or there could be a decision to continue treatment, which some carers would feel would not so much prolong her life as put off her inevitable death (Hammerman et al 1997). Worse still, for some carers, would be the continuation of aggressive treatment, which could result in the baby surviving with major morbidity. McHaffie (1998) suggests that the question that has evolved with time and experience is not *'Can* we save this baby?' but *'Should* we?'.

People often feel insecure about expressing their views to others who are perceived to have greater experience, in any area of life. One point that should be remembered is that length of experience does not automatically equate to volume or quality of experience. Also, if only those with a wealth of past experience take part in such decision-making, not only will inexperienced people never move forward, but neither will approaches to problems faced.

Christina will undoubtedly have an opinion, whether or not she wishes to express it. This opinion may be professionally formulated but influenced by personal values, beliefs and experiences. Alternatively, it is possible that she holds two opinions: one strictly formulated by her interpretation of professional rules and codes, the other arrived at by appeal to her fundamental values, beliefs and experiences as a human being. This could be why she can see two points of view. It can be very important that practitioners know where they stand on principles such as the value of life, the quality of life and the sanctity of life (see Further discussion), before they enter into a debate regarding the future treatment or non-treatment of any patient. Without this knowledge it is possible for people to be swayed by the persuasive articulation of others, rather than the rigour of the argument. In this case, someone could find themselves agreeing with everything that is said, however contradictory the points of view, rather than being able to balance the arguments to confirm or change their opinion. While it can be important to understand someone else's point of view, this does not mean that one has to agree with it. These points are well illustrated in Hazel McHaffie's novel *Holding On?* (McHaffie 1994).

Christina's role in the case conference will be the same as that of everyone else: they will all be there as advocates for Jasmine. Jasmine cannot put forward a view of her own; therefore, they should all put forward their views of what is in her best interests (UKCC 1992, 1996, 1999), as will her parents when requested. Miller (1996, pp. 124–125), in her discussion of the different decision-making approaches determined by Walters, suggests that there are limitations inherent in the 'best interests' approach. These limitations stem from the uncertain prognosis and lack of knowledge of what the child would want. Despite the limitations, this approach seems to be more just than any one of Walters' other approaches on its own: 'value of life', 'parental authority' or 'personhood'.

It has been stated by McHaffie & Fowlie (1996) that conflict some-times exists between medicine and nursing regarding both the aggressive treatment of neonates and the withdrawal of treatment. Christina's comfort in putting forward her views could depend on the attitude and chairpersonship of the neonatologist who has called the meeting. If the attitude is welcoming and not antagonistic of indi-vidual opinion, accepting and not condemning of differing views, then there is likely to be a more honest and fruitful debate.

QUESTION 2: CAN TREATMENT BE WITHHELD OR WITHDRAWN FROM JASMINE?

Initial thoughts on this question could be that treatment is often withheld while we 'watch and see' whether it becomes necessary, or withdrawn in favour of a different treatment, or when it is considered to be no longer of benefit. However, in this case, withholding could relate to resuscitation, and withdrawal could relate to current treat-ment, such as ventilation and artificial feeding, the intention being to allow Jasmine to die. Hence the discussion concerns the withholding or withdrawing of life-saving treatment and whether or not profes-sional carers are at liberty to do something that might result in death.

Some people would consider any action or non-action of this kind to be murder or manslaughter (Montgomery 1997). Others might use the term euthanasia, which could be viewed in a different light by some people as the intention is thought to be merciful as opposed to malicious. There could be debate as to whether it is active or passive euthanasia, depending on whether removal of equipment or treat-ment is seen as something active; also it would be involuntary as the baby could not consent to the action. However, causing the death of an individual is still considered to be illegal, and Montgomery (1997) explains that any distinction between the types of euthanasia is irrel-evant if it relates to a failure in the duty of care. Despite the perceived illegality, there have been cases where the judges have agreed to doctors withholding or withdrawing treatment. In Re C in 1989, the Judge agreed that the hospital should 'treat to die', ensur-ing that the baby was kept free of pain and distress (Mason & McCall Smith 1994). In the case of baby J (Mason & McCall Smith 1994), which was similar in some respects to that of Jasmine, Lord

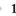

Donaldson determined that resuscitation need not take place in the case of further collapse, unless thought appropriate by the doctors at the time. He also made observations that could serve as guidance – not a ruling – for future cases. His statement maintained the position that usually action should be taken to prolong life, but that

> *...there will be cases in which ... it is not in the best interests of the child to subject it to treatment which will cause increased suffering and produce no commensurate benefit. (Nicholson 1990)*

Lord Donaldson stated that the person responsible for decision-making in the case should contemplate:

- *the assumed view of the patient;*
- *the prognosis in terms of pain and suffering – including the distress caused by any treatment;*
- *that the decision making was a co-operative effort between the doctors and parents* [or courts] *... on behalf of the child ... in his best interests;*
- *that any decision taken was one which would affect death by way of a side-effect ... withhold treatment designed to prevent death from natural causes. (Mason & McCall Smith 1994, pp 152–153)*

This last point suggests consideration of the doctrine of double effect, whereby someone would be judged according to the intention of their actions as opposed to the consequences of them (Aksoy 1999, Ferguson 1997). In Jasmine's case, this could be the removal of a treatment that was causing her pain or suffering; if she then died, the doctor would not be considered to have caused the death.

In the case of Airedale NHS Trust v Tony Bland (1993), Lord Goff suggested that decisions regarding withholding or withdrawing treatment should be viewed as in determining standards in the duty of care, according to the Bolam test; i.e. in accordance with: 'a responsible and competent body of relevant professional opinion' (Bolam v Friern HMC 1957). One of the difficulties here would be that different practices are carried out in different units.

The legal standpoint then, while not precise, does give some guidance and professional flexibility, but what about the ethical position? In view of the diversity of opinion held by society with regard to life and death decisions, particularly with regard to the issues surrounding the principles of value, quality and sanctity of life inherent in the euthanasia debate, it is unlikely that there will ever be one answer that is acceptable to all. As healthcare professionals, it is usual to seek ethical guidance from codes or guidelines produced by professional bodies. The *Code of Professional Conduct* (UKCC 1992) indicates the accountability of, in this case, the nurses and midwives with regard to acting in the interests of Jasmine (clauses 1 and 2), and to working within the professional team to provide appropriate care (clause 6). The doctors also have professional guidance. In 1997 the Royal College of Paediatrics and Child Health (RCPCH) produced *Withholding or Withdrawing Life Saving Treatment in Children. A Framework for Practice.* The foreword of this document states:

> *...Sometimes it is necessary to come to the conclusion that for an individual child – who might be a premature baby ... the more humane path is one of palliation, rather than a continuation of life-saving treatment ... our professional responsibilities do not allow us to walk away from such difficulties. (Baum 1997, p. 3)*

The document defines five situations where withholding or withdrawing treatment might be considered:

◆ The brain-dead child
◆ The permanent vegetative state
◆ The 'no chance' situation
◆ The 'no purpose' situation
◆ The 'unbearable' situation

It is possible that Jasmine could fit into any of the last three situations, each of which, in its own way, suggests that continued treatment is futile. However, Balfour-Lyn & Tasker (1996, p. 281) suggest that it is difficult to determine what futility is: it is not quantifiable as it 'encompasses a range of probabilities'. Gillon (1997, p. 339) also has concerns about the concept and states:

> *While it seems clear that doctors have no moral obligation to provide futile treatments and indeed where these are likely to cause burdens of one sort or another that they have a positive moral duty not to provide them, nonetheless futility judgements are so fraught with ambiguity, complexity and potential aggravation that they are best avoided altogether...*

The RCPCH document states that the House of Lords Select Committee on medical ethics received evidence from the British Paediatric Association (BPA) that 30% of neonatal deaths may have followed withdrawal of treatment. Jasmine's condition certainly fits into one of the categories of listed cases (RCPCH 1997). Withdrawal of treatment should not include withdrawal of palliative care and judges have emphasised that dignity and comfort should be paramount (McHaffie 1998).

A second, similar, document intended to assist doctors in such situations has been produced by the British Medical Association (BMA) (1999) *Withholding and Withdrawing Life-prolonging Medical Treatment. Guidance for Decision Making.* This document encourages doctors to balance the benefits and burdens to the patient, which is similar to considering the principles of beneficence (doing good) and non-maleficence (doing no harm). It is usually accepted that providing treatment and prolonging life would be good for the patient (in this case Jasmine), and that withholding or withdrawing treatment – allowing nature to take its course – would be harmful. However, it is possible that providing the treatment will result in greater or prolonged harm, with no good in sight (Geddes & Pace 1992, Miller 1996), suggesting that allowing Jasmine to die would be kinder.

QUESTION 3: WITH WHOM DOES THE FINAL DECISION REST?

In 1993 the Chief Medical Officer stated that policies regarding 'do not resuscitate' (DNR) orders were the responsibility of the consultant concerned (BMA & Royal College of Nursing 1993). This suggests that final life and death decisions rest with the consultants, keeping in mind that, where possible, patients should be involved in the decision-making. Obviously neonates are unable to take part in this process, so their parents are usually involved in decision-making on their behalf. This position has been supported in many legal cases. For instance, in the case of Re T (1997) before the Appeal Court, Judge Waite stated:

> ...the best interests of every child include an expectation that difficult decisions affecting the length and quality of life will be taken for it by the parent to whom its care has been entrusted by nature.

This case was about parental refusal of a liver transplant for their 18-month-old son, but the principle still applies to decisions regarding neonates. Judge Wilson, in Re C (1999), stated that in any application for a court order to act without parental consent the professionals' case would need to indicate positive grounds for overruling the parents. In this particular case, regarding the testing of a baby for human immunodeficiency virus, he found that the case was overwhelming.

McHaffie (1998, p. 386) highlights arguments for and against parental involvement:

The arguments for:
- ✦ *It is their right*
- ✦ *They have to live with the consequences*
- ✦ *Only they know their own breaking points*
- ✦ *They have different priorities which only they can represent*
- ✦ *A burden they choose to carry is better than one thrust upon them*

The arguments against:
- ✦ *They lack medical knowledge and understanding*
- ✦ *They are too emotionally stressed*
- ✦ *It is too onerous a burden for them to carry*
- ✦ *Their interests may conflict with those of the baby*
- ✦ *Their indecision may prolong the baby's suffering*
- ✦ *They have little precedent to guide them since they do not decide lesser things for their baby*

One of the arguments against parental involvement concerns a conflict of interests. Moral duties, professional codes of conduct and legal statements from relevant cases all suggest that the interests of the patient, in this case the baby, take precedence. However, some writers on dilemmas in neonatal care comment on the interests of the family (Grimley 1995, Miller 1996), and even society (Grimley 1995).

As stated above, the BPA suggests that 30% of neonatal deaths occur following withdrawal of treatment, but very few cases are taken to court for judicial rulings. This course of action would generally occur where the views of parents and professionals differ, as in the cases above. Other such cases in the 1990s have also received publicity.

In the case of Thomas Creedon, a severely brain damaged baby, the parents considered that his quality of life was so poor that artificial feeding should be withdrawn to allow him to die. The consultant, on the other hand, believed that all life should be valued, regardless of its condition, and the fact that Thomas could feel pain indicated that this was a life. He considered that feeding, even by artificial means, was a basic human right and should not be withdrawn. This case was due to go to court in 1996 but Thomas died from a chest infection which the general practitioner and parents chose not to treat (BBC 1996).

In New Zealand, Baby L's case was dealt with much earlier. Leaney Lavea was severely brain damaged. The doctors considered that treatment should be discontinued, but the parents could not accept the prognosis and took the case to court as they wished to continue treating her. The court's decision, with great respect for the value and quality of Leaney's life and respect for the family, was to discontinue treatment and allow the baby to die (BBC 1998).

However, in 1992 in Washington, USA, a woman chose to continue her pregnancy with an anencephalic fetus (McCarthy 1993). When Baby K was born, mechanical ventilation was required for respiratory distress. After a few days the doctors asked the mother for permission to issue a DNR order, but she refused on religious grounds, believing in the sanctity of life and that God would decide the fate of her daughter. After a year, which involved repeated ventilation and a total of four months in intensive care, the hospital sought a judicial ruling to withdraw treatment. The Judge ruled that discontinuation of treatment would amount to a discriminatory offence and that the mother had a right to insist on treatment; therefore, aggressive treatment had to continue.

Orr & Genesen (1997, p. 142) suggest that, in the USA at least, 'requests for inappropriate treatment' based on the belief in the sanctity of life are increasing. They also suggest that 'the most persistent requests … should be honoured'. This position appears to be upheld in a random survey of Danish residents (Norup 1998); however, McHaffie (1999) advises caution with regard to the use of such surveys as the responses are generally made based on little knowledge. In the UK, Dunn (1993) stated that he had only had one case where the parents had refused life-saving treatment for their baby, and this was on religious grounds. He had sought legal intervention and the treatment was carried out – an exchange transfusion. In the article, he stated:

I am still uncertain as to whether this action was ethically correct, even if it was medically justified. (Dunn 1993, p. 83)

In the conclusion of his discussion he states that the parents and doctors should make the decisions, in privacy, for the good of the baby. The BMA has also called for a less adversarial system (Dyer 1996) to deal with cases where doctors and parents disagree over what constitutes the best interests of the child.

Decision-making in neonatal care is all the more difficult because the patient is unable to engage in the process. Therefore, while case conferences involving all carers, professionals and parents may indicate a number of different views regarding any one baby, such as Jasmine, they surely must be the best way of producing the fullest picture on which to make a decision. Each person's input should be equally valued and a consensus could be reached (Richardson & Webber 1995); however, the consultant is still responsible for the final decision. Another alternative would be to have multidisciplinary clinical ethics committees in Trusts, where difficult cases could be discussed and courses of action determined objectively. This approach is supported by Great Ormond Street Hospital for Children (Larcher et al 1997). One cannot help but wonder, however, whether total objectivity is the most humane method of decision-making.

There have been cases where nurses or other healthcare workers have reported decisions or actions to appropriate authorities (Goff 1995). Consequently, even where parents and doctors have been in accord, these cases have been investigated and sometimes prosecutions have taken place. Although some people may wish to condemn these people for their interference, it should be realised that they are fulfilling their advocacy role as they believe they should, in cases where they report decisions before a death occurs. In cases where a death has already occurred, they are seeking to correct a moral and legal wrong. Nurses and midwives are directed to protect the interests of their patients or clients and to raise their concerns about appropriate care (UKCC 1992). If these professionals believe that the decisions or actions are not in the best interests of the patients, then they are duty bound to refer to another authority, although this course of action could cause great distress to all concerned.

FURTHER DISCUSSION

In discussing the questions above, the principles of value, quality and sanctity of life were raised. It would seem, from observations in classroom and clinical settings, that many people mention one of the principles while meaning all three. While they can undoubtedly be linked, these are separate principles and, as stated above, it can be important that practitioners know their own stance on them before becoming involved in life and death decision-making.

Value of life

Value generally equates to worth, and in the context of this chapter it is moral worth that is being considered, not financial worth. To consider that human beings are of moral worth suggests that they are all equal and should be treated as such (Harris 1985). There is much debate within sections of society regarding whether animals, or even plants, are of equal worth to human beings. To argue that this is not the case suggests that we must determine what it is that makes us so different that we can be considered of special worth.

The value of life is generally an extrinsic principle, although there is an intrinsic element. The intrinsic view can be highlighted by the statement: 'I value my life, therefore my life is valuable.' The extrinsic view, however, is more difficult. How is the value of someone else's life determined? According to Harris (1985, p. 7), many medical decisions 'presuppose particular answers to this question'. Harris states that abortion, of the type that we have come to know as 'social' can be acceptable only if the assumption is that the fetus is less valuable than the mother. Others might consider that acceptance of abortion, in these circumstances, has more to do with autonomy; however, this is his view and it amounts to 'competitive valuing'. Another example of this could be what occurs during any disaster – fire, flood, earthquake for instance. If decisions have to be made as to who to save, on what are these decisions based? As can be seen in all good disaster films at the cinema, aspects such as age, state of health, physical ability and usefulness in society may all feature in the decision-making. It could be argued that competitive valuing occurs regularly in health care, where so many people are competing for valuable resources. If a kidney becomes available for transplant and is deemed compatible for a six-year-old patient and a 60-year-old patient, difficult decisions have to be made, and this could occur based on such valuing. In many cases this subjective and unjust method of deciding has been superseded by more objective methods, which also create fierce debate (Cherry 1997), but which will not be discussed here.

Why should it be morally correct that, in one of the disasters mentioned above, most people – but by no means all – would save the humans before the animals? This is treating people as equals and as superior to other creatures; there are many who would be opposed to this view. However, the answer to this question would probably give us the answer regarding what it is that is so special about human beings. So, what is it that makes human life valuable? It is often accepted, by those who favour the view that human life has greater value than other forms of life, that 'personhood' is the key (Purdy & Tooley 1999, p. 36) and not the fact of being *Homo sapiens*. In other words, it is not just the fact that we were born human, but what it is that makes us persons. Harris (1985, pp. 16–17) considers that a person is

any being capable of valuing its own existence

which he suggests could be non-humans. Singer (cited in Toolis 1999) appears to agree with Harris, as he believes that many of the attributes of personhood are exhibited by other mammals and that, if the potential to personhood is put aside, then they are more worthy of consideration as persons than infants, particularly brain-damaged neonates. In Singer's view (cited in Cantor 1996, p. 1718), non-persons are:

…creatures with diminished rights and expectations, retaining some interests but lacking normal protection against involuntary death.

Harris' view is based on John Locke's late seventeenth century characterisation of a person as an intelligent, reflective and rational being who could think 'of itself in different times and places' (Harris 1985, p. 18). In Harris' view, this concept of the person has five functions:

1 *To enable us morally to distinguish between persons and animals, fish, plants and so on.*
2 *To have an account of the point at which, and the reasons why, the embryo or any live human tissue becomes valuable.*

3 *To recognise when and why human beings cease to be valuable or become less valuable than others.*

4 *To provide a framework that would in principle enable us to answer the question 'are there other people in the universe?'*

5 *To give us an account of what it is that is so great about ourselves.*

Neither Locke's nor Harris' considerations take account of unconscious or incompetent human beings, or neonates and infants. How old is someone likely to be before being able to 'value its own existence' or consider themself 'in different times and places'? Warnock (1998) has concerns regarding the classification of persons, generally because of the difficulties encountered with just such individuals.

Purdy & Tooley (1999) appear to have considered some of Locke's and Harris' anomalies when they proposed that personhood requires possession, current or past, of the following:

◆ the capacity to have a desire for continued existence
◆ the ability to be a continuing subject of experience and other mental states
◆ the capacity for self-consciousness

These properties appear to account for the fetus, neonate and infant, as the capacity or potential is there – it just needs time to develop. They also provide a framework to aid decision-making with regard to a person in a persistent vegetative state.

According to Mitchell (1990), the value of human life is a universal value that all societies appear to uphold to some extent. One reason is that a society with indifference to whether its members live or die would not survive. However, some societies have supported practices that some people would find barbaric, such as duelling, sacrificial killing and infanticide. Mitchell (1990, p. 35) also suggests that many societies have comparatively little regard 'for the value of lives of aliens and racial minorities'. By aliens he is referring to outsiders or foreigners, not extra-terrestrials. He questions the extent and reason why the value of human life is considered universal and his answer starts with the premise that most people want to live, and any moral system utilising the universalisation principle would include prohibition on killing. Prohibition of killing human beings, while there is no such ban on killing animals, suggests that human life is of greater value. Some people, however, do not want to live in some circumstances, so the value of life may not be acceptable as an absolute principle.

Mitchell (1990, p. 35) quotes Mahoney (1984), who eloquently described human life in a way appreciated by this author:

> *There is an element of sheer mystery about human existence which lays a claim upon men to reverence and respect it, to foster it and not to destroy it. Even on the most ordinary grounds, apart from any religious considerations, human life is a deep mystery ... at the heart of each one of us is an intractable, perhaps impenetrable, personal core.*

Quality of life

Generally, people understand what is meant by a 'quality' garment; it would include the fabric, cut, style, stitching, lining, etc. but what constitutes the quality of life? For some people it could be working hard and playing hard, filling all their spare time with activities: aerobics on Monday and Wednesday, swimming on Thursday, eating out with friends on Friday, rock climbing at the weekend. For others it might be the domestic bliss of parenting, homemaking, making children's costumes for the latest ballet venture, preparing for cub camp, curling up with a good book, or perhaps something else. These two examples are generally lifestyles as opposed to life. For quality in life itself, people quote factors that include: good health, to love and be loved, maintainance of mobility, retention of all faculties, sometimes even wealth.

Quality is a personal, subjective notion; it is therefore intrinsic. We can only guess with regard to quality in someone else's life, and that would be based on our own values, beliefs, attitudes and experiences. It would be difficult to determine the quality of life in the case of an adult, so it would be more difficult in the case of a neonate, when it is future quality that is being considered. Mitchell (1990) suggests that, in cases where our reflective judgement indicates that a neonate's life should not be prolonged, looking for a rationale creates a dilemma. On the one hand we can consider the quality of life, which in itself is a difficult task. Alternatively, there is the cost–benefit analysis, that is whether the benefit of the treatment to the baby outweighs the costs to it in terms of risk or pain; this can also be difficult to determine. Muldoon et al (1998) agree that burdensome factors should be taken into account. They also state that the quality of life includes objective functioning and subjective well-being. Their 'operational definitions', however, could not be applied to a brain-damaged neonate and are, therefore, not particularly useful in the case of Jasmine. There could also be a further dimension to decision-making in such cases, that is the availability of resources. However, it is unlikely that many professionals would be prepared to give lack of resources, especially finance, as a rationale to discontinue life support. It is more likely that quality of life or the cost–benefit analysis for the neonate would be stated – whether completely true or not.

Sanctity of life

The sanctity of life principle stems from the religious view that all human life is sacred; however, religion is not the only source of moral guidance. Rational determination of rights and wrongs, as the foundation of ethical codes, guides the moral attitudes of many non-religious people. However, according to Kuhse & Singer (1985), removal of the principle of the sanctity of life from the religious framework weakens the principle itself.

There is generally no question that people have the right to life, supported by the *Human Rights Act 1998*, but is life as they would experience it what they would want if they could choose (e.g. people in a persistent vegetative state or anencephalics)? A television documentary, some years ago, focussed on an anencephalic child, about two years old, with brainstem function only. She had no consciousness or thought in any way and she was being kept 'alive' by parenteral nutrition. Although it could be said that she did not know of anything different, we have to consider whether any two year old would choose to be in that state.

According to Glover (1988, p. 41):

> *To say taking life is always wrong commits us to absolute pacifism.*
> *But clearly a pacifist and non-pacifist can share the view that*
> *killing is in itself an evil. They need only differ with regard to*
> *when, if ever, killing is permissible to avoid other evils. It is better*
> *to say that taking a life is directly wrong ...*

It is possible to believe that killing is only directly wrong (i.e. wrong in itself) when the person does not want to die, or where the years of which he or she is deprived would have been generally happy ones. Glover also suggests that the doctrine of the sanctity of life is unacceptable, but that the embedded moral view (that it is normally directly wrong – that in most cases to take a life in the absence of harmful side-effects is wrong) should be retained.

Glover's (1988, p. 138) alternative view to the sanctity of life is that there are two objections to killing, other than any inherent side-effects or pain:

> *it is wrong to reduce the amount of worthwhile life* [but worthwhile to whom?]*;*
> *it is wrong to override someone's autonomy when he wants to go on living.*

The principle of the sanctity of life is commonly combined with the doctrines of 'double effect' and 'acts and omissions'; these temper the severity of the principle and therefore prevent us from being committed to taking all possible positive steps to save lives, however terrible the state of them. Warnock (1998), however, cautions against the diluting of the sanctity of life as she sees it as a slippery slope situation. If we agree to allow death in situations such as Jasmine's, she wonders whether the slope will lead us to an 'ethical quagmire' where we encourage the death of the helpless and those requiring the use of significant resources.

Cases, where we would predict that the quality of life is so poor that it would be better for the person not to be alive show that the traditional sanctity of human life principle does not relieve us of the burden of decision-making in difficult situations; the principles of beneficence and non-maleficence must enter the frame. Unless such decisions are computerised, personal judgement cannot be avoided.

These statements from McCormick (cited in Weir 1984), although old in origin, appear to bring together the three principles of value, quality and sanctity of life in a humane and sensible way:

> *...every human being, regardless of age or condition, is of incalculable worth*

but he feels that:

> *...it is wrong to preserve the life of one with no capacity for those aspects of life that we regard as human.*

Killing or letting die?

Discussions with many healthcare professionals suggest that most of them consider that there is a definite difference between killing and letting die. However, if we take a consequentialist approach to the question and consider the consequences of both killing and letting die, the result in both cases would be death. This could suggest that there is no difference and that healthcare professionals convince themselves that there is a difference because it suits their purpose, which is to allow certain patients to die instead of inflicting continued life. If this stance is correct, then it could be deemed just as immoral and illegal to allow a baby such as Jasmine to die, as it would be to take active steps to end her life (Johnson 1993, Randall 1997).

The opposite view could be taken of course, still maintaining that there is no difference between killing and letting die: if it is deemed moral and legal to let her die, then it should also be moral and legal to bring her life to an end to prevent any further suffering. Singer is reported to hold this view. He considers that selective infanticide of disabled children is justified if the parents consider that continuation of that life would badly affect their happiness (Toolis 1999).

It is often considered that killing requires an action and letting die requires no action, as with active and passive euthanasia. This is often referred to as the acts and omissions doctrine. It should be remembered that both acts and omissions can be positive and negative. An action can be morally or professionally right, and therefore positive, or it can be morally or professionally wrong and therefore negative. An omission is often thought of as something that someone neglected to do, making it negative, whereas it could be something someone chose not to do, rightly or wrongly, making it positive or negative respectively. For instance, if a young man has a head injury, treatment for which would mean a full recovery, but medical staff do nothing, would his death be equivalent to killing or letting die? Leaving aside the civil tort of negligence, this might be considered to be a case of killing by non-action and, therefore, manslaughter.

If we accept the notion that killing requires an action and letting die requires non-action, it suggests that withholding life-saving treatment is equivalent to letting die, whilst withdrawing such treatment would equate to killing. This was not the view held by the Court of

Appeal in the Tony Bland case (Airedale NHS Trust v Bland 1993), where it was agreed that feeding could be stopped and he could be allowed to die. The ruling did, however, make a distinction between withdrawing treatment to allow death and taking active steps to cause death (Johnson 1993).

Sugarman et al (1996), in their consideration of the moral defensibility of withholding or withdrawing treatment, indicate three perspectives. The first suggests that, in a medical crisis, action should be taken and treatment commenced until such time as the treatments prove ineffective. This would make withdrawal of such treatment defensible as all reasonable efforts had been made. The second perspective suggests that withholding treatment is more defensible as it prevents the complications that could be caused by the treatment, and withdrawing treatment puts the professionals in the position of carrying out an act as opposed to an omission. The third approach was, as stated above, that they are morally equivalent.

Ethical arguments can be made for and against the withholding and withdrawing of life-saving treatment. However, based on their research into life and death decision-making in neonatal practice, McHaffie & Fowlie (1996, p. 8) make the following observation:

> For the clinician caught up in the human tragedy of these choices there is a very real difference between theoretical ethics and clinical ethics ... What may seem a perfectly logical argument in the lecture theatre or in an academic paper, assumes quite different proportions in the face of infant suffering or parental grief or actual medical responsibility.

Decision-making may be based on the distinction between what is perceived as ordinary and extraordinary means; however, this in itself may be difficult to determine. For instance, use of mechanical ventilation may be considered by some to be an extraordinary means, but, where the infant cannot breathe for itself at all, it could be considered ordinary. A particularly contentious issue is that of feeding, whereby some practitioners consider all forms of feeding and hydration to be basic care and, therefore, non-negotiable in terms of discontinuation. Others consider that offering feeds for the baby to take or not take is basic care, but to tube feed is part of treatment and therefore can be considered for discontinuation. Where this decision is made it is legal for nurses and midwives to follow the instructions, but they have the difficult task of day-to-day care of the baby and dealing with parental anxieties (Miller 1996). In some cases oral feeds might be offered for comfort – possibly the comfort of staff and relatives.

The *Human Rights Act 1998* (part 1, article 2) includes the right to life:

> *Everyone's right to life shall be protected by law ...*

but perhaps this refers to life as that individual wishes to live it. In the case of Jasmine, a severely brain-damaged neonate, those concerned can use only their intuition and experience, as parents and professionals, to guess what she would want.

APPLYING THE THEORIES TO JASMINE'S CASE

Utilitarian views

It is possible that both act- and rule-utilitarians, in consideration of the greatest good for all involved directly, and society as a whole with regard to resources, would support both the withholding and withdrawing of treatment.

Deontological views

A Kantian, although unable to use autonomy directly, would consider the 'means to a end' aspect. If Jasmine was allowed to die for the sake of the family's interests or for lack of resources, then it would be an immoral act. If it is thought to be in her best interests, then it would possibly be considered until universalisation was applied, as it would be judged immoral to allow all babies to die. Even if the universalisation was narrowed down to all brain-damaged babies, it would still be immoral to allow them all to die. It is possible that withholding treatment could be accepted, whereas withdrawing treatment would not.

Traditional deontologists would be unlikely to support either withholding or withdrawing treatment, because of the sanctity of life principle.

Pluralists would order the duties in accordance with the case. It is probable that non-maleficence, beneficence and justice would hold the priorities. While justice would require them to consider whether a brain-damaged baby should be treated differently from any other baby, the other principles may well lead them towards withholding treatment and possibly the withdrawal of the most invasive or painful treatments.

REFERENCES

Airedale NHS Trust v Bland 1993 1 All E R 821

Askoy S 1999 Is the intention relevant to whether an act is morally right or wrong in medical practice? Bulletin of Medical Ethics 151:21–24

Balfour-Lyn I M, Tasker R C 1996 Futility and death in paediatric medical intensive care. Journal of Medical Ethics 22:279–281

Baum D 1997 Foreword. In: Withholding or withdrawing life saving treatment in children. A framework for practice. Royal College of Paediatrics and Child health, London

BBC 1996 Panorama: a life in limbo – Thomas Creedon. BBC, London

BBC 1998 Heart of the Matter: one brief life – Leaney Lavea. BBC, London

British Medical Association & Royal College of Nursing 1993 Cardiopulmonary resuscitation – a statement. BMJ & RCN, London

British Medical Association 1999 Withholding and withdrawing life-prolonging medical treatment. Guidance for decision making. BMJ, London

Bolam v Friern HMC 1957 2 All E R 118

Cantor N L 1996 Rethinking life and death. Michigan Law Review 94(6):1718–1738

Cherry C 1997 Health care, human worth and the limits of the particular. Journal of Medical Ethics 23:310–314

Dunn P M 1993 Appropriate care of the newborn: ethical dilemmas. Journal of Medical Ethics 19:82–84

Dyer C 1996 Mother wins right to refuse treatment for her child. British Medical Journal 313:1101

Ferguson P R 1997 Causing death or allowing to die? Developments in the law. Journal of Medical Ethics 23:368–372

Geddes S, Pace N 1992 Selectively withholding treatment from newborn babies. British Journal of Hospital Medicine, 47(4):481–484

Gillon R 1997 Futility – too ambiguous and pejorative a term? Journal of Medical Ethics 23:339–340

Glover J 1988 Causing death and saving lives. Penguin Books, London

Goff R 1995 A matter of life and death. Medical Law Review 3(1):1–21

Grimley I 1995 Dilemmas of care. Nursing Times 91(18):42–43

Hammerman C, Kornbluth E, Lavie O, Zadka P, Aboulafia Y, Eidelman A 1997 Decision-making in the critically ill neonate: cultural background v individual life experiences. Journal of Medical Ethics 23:164–169

Harris J 1985 The value of life. Routledge, London

Johnson K 1993 A moral dilemma: killing and letting die. British Journal of Nursing, 2(12):635–640

Kuhse H, Singer P 1985 Should the baby live? Oxford University Press, Oxford

Larcher V F, Lask B, McCarthy M 1997 Paediatrics at the cutting edge: do we need clinical ethics committees? Journal of Medical Ethics 23:245–249

McCarthy M 1993 Anencephalic baby's right to life? Lancet 342:919

McHaffie H E 1994 Holding on? Books for Midwives Press, Hale, UK

McHaffie H E 1998 Withdrawing treatment from neonates: a review of the issues. British Journal of Midwifery 6(6):384–386

McHaffie H E 1999 Treatment of extremely premature newborns: a survey of attitudes among Danish physicians. Midwives Information & Resource Service 9(1):102 (abstract comments).

McHaffie H E, Fowlie P W 1996 Life, death and decisions. Hochland & Hochland, Hale, UK

Mahoney J 1984 Bioethics and belief: religion and medicine in dialogue. Sheed & Ward, London

Mason J K, McCall Smith R A 1994 Law and medical ethics. Butterworths, London

Miller P 1996 Ethical issues in neonatal intensive care. In: Frith L (ed) Ethics and midwifery. Issues in contemporary practice. Butterworth Heinemann, Oxford

Mitchell B 1990 The value of human life. In: Byrne P (ed) Medicine, medical ethics and the value of life. John Wiley, Chichester

Montgomery 1997 Health care law. Oxford University Press, Oxford

Muldoon M F, Barger S D, Flory J D, Manuck S B 1998 What are quality of life measurements measuring? British Medical Journal 316:542–544

Nicholson R (ed) 1990 Court permits doctors not to resuscitate gravely handicapped infant. Bulletin of Medical Ethics 63:22–23

Norup M 1998 Limits of neonatal treatment: a survey of attitudes in the Danish population. Journal of Medical Ethics 24:200–206

Orr R D, Genesen L B 1997 Requests for 'inappropriate' treatment based on religious beliefs. Journal of Medical Ethics 23:142–147

Purdy L, Tooley M 1999 Is abortion murder? In: Palmer M (ed) Moral problems in medicine. Lutterworth, Cambridge

Randall F 1997 Why causing death is not necessarily morally equivalent to allowing to die – a response to Ferguson. Journal of Medical Ethics 23:373–376

Re C (a child) 1999 Infant must have HIV test. Bulletin of Medical Ethics 151:7–8

Re T (wardship: medical treatment) 1997 1 FLR 502

Richardson J, Webber I 1995 Ethical issues in child health care, Mosby, London

Royal College of Paediatrics & Child Health 1997 Withholding or withdrawing life saving treatment in children. A framework for practice. RCPCH, London

Sugarman B, Montvilo R K, Matarese C J 1996 Neonatal euthanasia: attributions of students and nurses. Journal of Social Issues 52(2):189–196

Toolis K 1999 The most dangerous man in the world. Guardian Weekend 6 November: 52–55

UKCC 1992 Code of professional conduct. UKCC, London

UKCC 1996 Guidelines for professional practice. UKCC, London

UKCC 1999 Practitioner–client relationships and the prevention of abuse. UKCC, London

Warnock M 1998 An intelligent person's guide to ethics. Duckworth, London

Weir R 1984 Selective nontreatment of handicapped newborns. Oxford University Press, New York

SUGGESTED ADDITIONAL READING

Dimond B 1996 The legal aspects of child heath care. Mosby, London

Gillon R 1986 Philosophical medical ethics. John Wiley, Chichester

Perrens C 1996 A parent's dilemma. Paediatric Nursing 8(7):18–19

Stanley J M 1992 Part III: Decisions involving neonates and other patients who have never achieved decision-making capacity. Journal of Medical Ethics 18:13–15

Wright S 1993 What makes a person? Nursing Times 89(21):42–45

11

Conclusion

The modern midwife qualifies at a different academic level to her more experienced colleagues. She is able to analyse, synthesise and evaluate the care that is offered to women and babies. This makes her more academically able to be proactive and challenging within the multidisciplinary team – once she has developed her assertiveness. When she has developed her expertise through experience, this makes her a worthy advocate for women, babies and the midwifery profession. This is not to say that her more experienced colleagues are not capable of utilising such skills. On the contrary, some such midwives have developed the cognitive skills without the assistance of educational programmes designed to help them. Some others have undertaken post-registration education in midwifery, women's health or other relevant subjects. In both pre- and post-registration courses, in this author's experience, education in ethics and law seems to make a real difference to the way in which these practitioners function; they appear to view practice through different eyes.

This second edition of *Ethics in Midwifery* has aimed to maintain the general approach of the first edition, while trying to increase the application to issues in practice. Chapters 1 and 2, as before but updated and slightly expanded in places, explain what ethics is, what a moral dilemma is, and how one can attempt to resolve it. Major theories have been explained and there has been the suggestion that, while it is important to know the theories in order to understand how and why others make their decisions, perhaps there is another way.

Chapter 3 is a new chapter, intended as a bridge between the theoretical chapters in Section 1 and the application to practice, by considering the ethical dimensions of midwifery. Section 2 includes six new case studies, some dealing with the principles considered in the previous edition, but through the vehicle of different situations. There are also some totally new cases which deal with more contemporary issues. What the reader will have discovered is the increase in the application of law. Civil law, as previously mentioned, is underpinned by ethics and it is often inappropriate to separate the two disciplines. Practitioners need to be able to see how they can be interlinked as well as how they can be separated.

Midwives need to be able to recognise moral conflicts and dilemmas; they also need to be able to draw on the relevant principles with which to solve them. If they are unsure about which, if any, major theory they wish to follow, my general advice would be in keeping with that of Walt Disney's character – Jiminy Cricket:

Always let your conscience be your guide.
(Washington & Harline 1940, Bourne)

Glossary

act-utilitarianism The traditional form of utilitarianism where every single action is judged by its consequences

autonomy The capacity to be rational and in control of liberty and freedom

battery A term in criminal law for any physical contact without prior consent

beneficence To do good or to help, as in doctors' duty to their patients

casuistry Disentanglement and re-ordering of 'duties' in conflict

categorical imperative This is Kant's guidance on objective moral action, where it is decided what you ought to want and you should be happy with it

conflict (moral) A trial of strength between principles

deontology An ethical theory based on duty

descriptivism The view that moral judgements have descriptive meaning only

dilemma A problem created by the conflict of principles, where all the choices offered seem to lack total satisfaction

emotivism A theory concerned with the meaning of ethical terms

ethics The underlying reasons, or set of standards, that regulate behaviour

implied consent The assumption that certain positive actions indicate acceptance by the recipient

informed consent The uncoerced permission given by an individual, following consideration of sufficient information, for another to take action

liberty   Having the right to do as you please

licensing authority   The Human Fertilisation and Embryology Authority (HFEA), responsible for the issuing of licenses for treatment, storage and research in connection with activities covered by the Act

monism   A theory based on one supreme principle or duty

moral   Relates to the rights and wrongs of everyday living

negligence   A breach in the duty of care that may or may not be proved to have caused the harm or injury in question

non-maleficence   To do no harm

particularism   A belief in the development of moral sensibilities rather than reliance on formal theories

paternalism   Making decisions on behalf of those who are rational enough to make their own decisions

pluralism   A theory based on more than one principle, with none being supreme

prima-facie duties   A method of prioritising specific duties

quality of life   The intrinsically determined attributes that make life worth living; extrinsic determination is mainly by guesswork

rational   Self-determining, self-controlled

rule-utilitarianism   A modification of act-utilitarianism, it assesses an act according to moral rules

sanctity of life   The belief that life is sacred

subjectivist   Someone who believes that moral attitudes are a matter of taste

teleological   A doctrine that considers everything to have been created by God to serve humankind

universalisability   A principle that tests the morality of a judgement by universalising it

utilitarianism   A theory based on the consequences of actions

value of life   The worth placed on human life, sometimes intrinsically but usually extrinsically

Index of authors

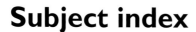

Subject index